NHA Phlebotomy Study Guide 2025-2026

Complete Review + 480 Questions and Detailed Answer Explanations for the Certified Phlebotomy Technician Exam (4 Full-Length Exams)

Table of Contents

Introduction

This study guide is your handy companion while preparing for the NHA CPT Examinations. This guide serves only to supplement your existing knowledge. You should always still refer to your textbooks to provide a deeper understanding of the topics outlined here.

Phlebotomy traditionally referred to the act of taking blood from a vein for laboratory testing. It has now evolved to refer to a special department in the hospital, apart from the usual nurses and medical technologists. With this evolution, national certifications have been instituted to assure the public of the skills and qualifications of every health care professional. Hence, the NHA CPT exam.

NHA CPT Examination

This examination covers 100 scored multiple-choice questions and 20 unscored items over a time period of 120 minutes. It assesses the aspiring phlebotomist in five general domains. These are:

- Safety and compliance
- Patient preparation
- Routine blood collection
- Special collection
- Processing

Registration

The first step to becoming a certified phlebotomist is registering online with the National Healthcareer Association. You can find the specific steps on the NHA website.

Scheduling

Next, you will need to schedule your examination through NHA portals via telephone or the internet. After successfully scheduling an examination, wait for the confirmation email. This contains your test date, time and testing site address.

In addition to in-person exams, NHA offers a remote online examination. You will need to use a compatible system with a microphone and video camera. The test runs on the Google Chrome browser.

Cancellation and Missed Examination

You are allowed to cancel the examination at least 24 hours before your scheduled test. Otherwise, failing to show up or arriving late will forfeit your examination fee.

In-Person Examination

You should arrive at the testing site 30 minutes before your scheduled time. The testing site has extensive security measures. You are expected to conduct yourself in a professional manner. Personal items, coats and hats must be deposited at the security check sites.

You will not be allowed to eat, drink or smoke at the testing site.

Take a valid, signed government-issued photo ID card. The name on the card must match the name you used to register for the exam. Failing to present a valid ID card renders your examination invalid and forfeits your examination fee.

After going through the security check, you will be directed to the test center's computer and given 15 minutes to complete a tutorial. This is not counted in your total examination time. Make the most of this time to familiarize yourself with the system. Sample questions are provided. These do not count toward your test score.

You will be provided with a pencil and two pieces of paper for notes.

Remote Online Examination

For remote examinations, a proctor will be assigned to you. They will monitor your actions on screen. Interruptions, unauthorized actions or people on video or audio will result in the proctor pausing your examination.

Interruptions that are not corrected appropriately may result in the proctor canceling your test.

Have a valid, signed government-issued photo ID card to show to the proctor. The name on the card must match the name you used to register for the exam. Failing to present a valid ID card renders your examination invalid and forfeits your examination fee.

You can launch the examination 30 minutes before the scheduled time. You are allowed to use two pieces of paper for notes during the examination. You are required to show both sides of these to the proctor. You will need to tear these up in front of your proctor at the end of the examination. You are not permitted to take breaks during the examination.

Examination Result

After successfully completing your examination, you will receive an email that explains how you will receive your test scores.

Retake Guidelines

If you fail the examination, you will be given two more chances. You will need to repeat the registration and scheduling processes. You must wait at least 30 days before each attempt.

A third attempt and each subsequent attempt after this is allowed only after waiting one year.

Chapter 1: The Phlebotomy Professional

The Phlebotomist

Phlebotomy traditionally referred to the act of taking blood from a vein for laboratory testing. Since then, health care has evolved. Health care workers are now being cross-trained to perform interdisciplinary procedures to follow a more patient-centered approach. A few years ago, laboratory staff took turns making rounds around the hospital to perform venipuncture and returned to the laboratory to process the specimens. This was time-consuming. As a solution, phlebotomy was decentralized. Phlebotomy now refers to a special department in the hospital, apart from the usual nursing staff and medical technologists.

Roles of the Phlebotomist

Once you receive your certification, you will take on the role of a phlebotomist, a crucial player on the health care team. You will not simply take blood. You must perform technical and clerical functions and display good interpersonal skills.

Your duties include:

1. Ensuring that you have the right patient for whom the test is indicated.
2. Collecting the right specimen.
3. Selecting the correct specimen tubes.
4. Properly labeling all containers with the needed information.
5. Handling and transporting specimens in a timely fashion.
6. Processing specimens before distributing them to the appropriate laboratory sections.
7. Creating appropriate electronic records.
8. Interacting effectively with patients and other hospital workers.
9. Keeping confidentiality guidelines and abiding by Health Insurance Portability and Accountability (HIPAA) rules on patient information.
10. Observing all safety precautions, quality control and waste disposal procedures.
11. Keeping up with phlebotomy education programs.

Additionally, you may be assigned to other tasks by your supervisors, such as:

1. Teaching phlebotomy skills to other health care workers.
2. Monitoring specimen quality.
3. Evaluating existing guidelines and protocols for specimen collection.
4. Performing additional tasks related to patient care, such as electrocardiograms, taking vital signs, point-of-care testing or assisting physicians with lumbar punctures.

Phlebotomists may be employed in areas other than hospitals, such as:

1. Physician offices or a physician group laboratory
2. Health Management Organizations (HMOs)
3. Government clinics
4. Reference laboratories
5. Home health care units
6. Off-site clinics

Professional Traits of the Phlebotomist

In the health care setting, you are expected to act professionally. You, as a professional phlebotomist, are expected to be:

Dependable and Responsible

Diagnostic testing can be done only if a specimen is properly collected. Your role in health care delivery is crucial. Certain specimens are time dependent, and some are collected at intervals. You should be dependable enough not to miss STAT and timed collections.

Committed and Cooperative

Working in the health care field can be stressful. Often it is unpredictable, and emergencies can occur. Patients rely on a fully committed health care staff that collaborates during such situations. As a phlebotomist, you are part of this team. Show your commitment and cooperation by attending staff meetings and keeping up with the latest policies.

Honest and Dignified

Display integrity by admitting your faults. This could be crucial to a patient's safety.

Compassionate and Polite

Most of your duties center around patients. Always be aware that they are often sick and anxious. Practice empathy when dealing with their concerns and try to reassure them.

Always introduce yourself before you approach patients.

You may encounter patients' relatives as well. Extending courtesy to them demonstrates your compassion.

Competent and Organized

Avoid overconfidence. Do not attempt procedures you are not yet familiar with. Never hesitate to ask your colleagues if you are uncertain about something.

Having a well-organized workspace displays competence.

Each laboratory request is prioritized according to the physician's requirements. It can be routine, ASAP, STAT or timed.

A **routine** sample is preferably collected during the basal state early in the day. It may be collected throughout the day as well. Facilities may schedule their phlebotomists to carry out collections at certain times during the day.

ASAP stands for "as soon as possible," while a **STAT** test requires an immediate collection and analysis. STAT is given the highest priority. These requests often come from emergency departments or critical care units.

A **timed** specimen may be requested to evaluate the body's metabolic functions (such as in glucose tolerance testing and drug monitoring). For these tests, appropriate timing is crucial to provide physicians with a picture of the patient's metabolism of the compounds.

A crucial component of your duties as a phlebotomist involves organizing your time and schedule to accommodate these special collections.

Dressed Appropriately

A neat and clean appearance creates an impression of professionalism.

Follow the guidelines set by your facility. In general, this includes a clean lab coat and conservative clothing.

Dangling jewelry; long, unkempt hair; and long artificial nails should be avoided.

Communicating Effectively

This involves the interplay of three skills:

- **Verbal communication**, including tone of voice and choice of words
- **Listening** attentively
- **Nonverbal communication**, including body language

Age and educational achievement, hearing loss, language and emotions may be **barriers to verbal communication**. These may be overcome by:

- Avoiding the use of medical jargon
- Using age-appropriate words when speaking to children
- Speaking clearly and looking at the patient while speaking
- Using hand signals for patients who are hard of hearing
- Asking for the assistance of an interpreter for patients who cannot speak English
- Speaking calmly and reassuring anxious patients

While communication mainly involves language, its primary component is nonverbal.

You will interact with a patient for only a few minutes, but the way you walk and carry yourself will leave a message. Smiling and maintaining eye contact helps patients feel at ease with you. This facilitates effective communication and builds trust.

Conversely, seeming distracted and not looking at the patient gives the impression of disinterest, unease and incompetence.

Respectful of Cultural Diversity

Respecting cultural diversity aids in communication and demonstrates professionalism. It spans more than just language barriers. It includes differences in customs and values that affect the interactions between the phlebotomist and the patient.

Always be alert to your patients' reactions when you approach them, and be sensitive to their culture.

For example, a Muslim woman or her husband may not allow a male phlebotomist to extract her blood. Asking politely first and accommodating their culture will demonstrate professionalism.

Legal and Ethical Considerations

The principles of an individual's professional and personal conduct are governed by ethical codes. These determine how to act correctly and carry out your daily activities concerning the boundaries and rights of other people. In many instances, the right actions may not be obvious. Learning these principles helps you make the right decisions during difficult situations.

For example, a worried son confronts you at the door to the patient's room. He wants to know his mother's diagnosis. You are not authorized to disclose this information to anyone without the patient's written consent.

Sometimes, it may not be so simple.

Bioethical principles governing health care include the following.

Autonomy

Patients have the right to decide what to do with their bodies. They can consent to or refuse any procedure.

When a patient refuses to have blood extracted, you can try to explain the need and the procedure, but you cannot impose on the person's right to autonomy. In court, forcing a procedure, even for the patient's good, is viewed as physical battery. In this situation, respect the patient's decision. Inform the nurses and document the patient's refusal.

Nonmaleficence

This means to do no harm. With every medical procedure or diagnostic test, there is always a risk of harm. Harm must be avoided whenever possible.

Beneficence

You must keep the patient's best interest in mind at every encounter.

Informed Consent

The patient has the right to know the risks and benefits before any procedure.

Express consent

This is primarily reserved for invasive procedures, such as surgery or lumbar punctures, when the patient is required to express consent through writing.

Verbal consent is also acceptable, but it is less safe. It is prudent to document verbal consent in the patient's chart.

Implied Consent

This is common with venipuncture procedures. You explain how you will perform the venipuncture, informing patients that this was ordered by their physician. The patients assume your competence and allow you to proceed by extending their arms.

Consent is also assumed for emergency treatments.

Consent for Children and Incapacitated Patients

Procedures for children, comatose patients and cognitively impaired patients require their parents' or legal caregiver's consent.

In some situations, judicial courts may need to give the final ruling.

Consent for HIV tests

The rules for HIV testing may vary by state, depending on the existing laws. Always keep updated with the HIV consent protocol of your state.

Opt-out screening is a procedure in which patients (aged 13 to 64 years old) are informed of the HIV screening procedure as a part of routine care. Patients are given a chance to ask questions or decline.

In certain states, during an accidental needlestick to a medical professional, a physician may order HIV testing without the patient's consent. This is done to protect the medical professional's health. However, the results cannot be documented in the patient's chart.

Tort Law

A **tort** is an act of causing harm to another person or their property. It may or may not be intentional. Negligence is generally considered unintentional.

Assault refers to touching another person or threatening to do so without their consent. For example, when dealing with an irate patient, the phlebotomist threatens to hold the individual down to extract blood.

Battery is the act of causing harm to another person. Surgeons performing additional procedures without express consent may be charged with battery. For example, a surgeon finds and removes an ovarian tumor during an appendectomy. The patient consented only to the appendectomy. Therefore, the surgeon may be liable.

Defamation refers to acts that may cause harm to reputation. It may be verbal or in writing. This also pertains to breaches of confidentiality.

Libel is the act of publishing false, defamatory content.

Slander is saying false and malicious words.

Invasion of privacy is encroaching on another's right to be kept from public exposure. Releasing confidential data to unauthorized persons and entering patient wards without authorization are examples of invasion of privacy.

Malpractice

In the clinical sense, **malpractice** refers to a medical professional's misconduct or error, which results in injury or compromise to a patient.

Situations that phlebotomists must avoid:

1. Collecting crossmatched specimens from the wrong patient. This results in a hemolytic transfusion reaction and renal failure, which requires hemodialysis.

2. Probing vigorously, causing hematoma. This enlarges to compress the brachial nerve. The patient loses function in the affected arm.

Negligence is defined as failure to provide reasonable care, subject to the standards of care. The phlebotomist is subject to Clinical Laboratory Improvement Amendments (CLIA) standards.

Note that forgetting to return the bed rails after extracting blood, causing the patient to fall and sustain injuries, is a potential lawsuit.

To avoid these situations, you must consistently abide by the procedures and standards of care according to the Clinical and Laboratory Standards Institute (CLSI) and CLIA.

Risk Management

With every procedure, there is a potential risk of injury. You should take every precaution to mitigate the risks.

Risk management aims to develop protocols to protect everyone (patients and health care staff) from preventable harm. Even employers are protected, as it helps them avoid substantial costs these harms might accrue.

Risk management programs determine the risks and then develop policies to prevent them. Subsequently, they educate the staff and patients. They continually evaluate the programs and enact improvements when needed.

The **incident report** allows a witness to describe an incident and the actions taken to correct it. The report documents the incident and the investigation.

A **sentinel event** refers to an unexpected severe injury, often leading to death in the context of health care provision. These events include medication errors, retained foreign material following surgery, falls, assault, surgery on the wrong site and treatment delays.

These protocols are continually improving. It is therefore important that all staff be informed effectively.

Health Insurance Portability and Accountability Act (HIPAA)

This federal legislation covers many health care issues beyond the scope of the laboratory setting.

It was primarily created for the following reasons:

- To allow employees with preexisting medical conditions to enroll in health insurance
- To detect fraud more easily
- To improve efficiency by utilizing electronic records
- To safeguard confidentiality

Patients expect the highest level of confidentiality from their health providers. This is rule number one in the clinical setting. Patient information must remain protected. It can be discussed only on a need-to-know basis. Personal health information is protected by HIPAA.

As outlined in HIPAA, all health care providers, including you as a phlebotomist, must obtain patients' written consent to share their information.

By releasing patient information to the patient's relatives or fellow health care workers or inappropriately accessing the electronic records, you can be charged with violating HIPAA. These consequences may range from suspension to imprisonment. You may even be charged with defamation for breaching a patient's confidentiality.

You will be assigned to collect sensitive specimens, such as for HIV screening and sexually transmitted diseases, as well as drug screening. Discussing such sensitive information breaches confidentiality. Be careful when posting photos or information on social media as well.

Operational Regulatory Standards

Clinical and Laboratory Standards Institute (CLSI)

This agency develops a set of standards by which every laboratory procedure is measured. Should there be any legal proceedings, the regulations outlined in CLSI describe the proper procedures that should have been followed.

The Joint Commission

This commission takes charge of accrediting health care institutions across the United States, intending to continually improve health care quality. Every two years, a survey team visits laboratories to assess their adherence to the National Patient Safety Goals and renew their accreditation.

The **National Patient Safety Goals** include a two-method verification for accurately identifying the patient.
Patient identifiers include:

- First name and last name
- Patient ID number
- Date of birth
    - Labeling specimen containers while the patient is around.
    - Taking note that the patient's room number and ward do not qualify as reliable identifiers
    - Efficient communication systems
    - Informing the right staff of critical values
    - Taking standard precautions to mitigate risks of infections
    - Adherence to hand hygiene protocols

Clinical Laboratory Improvement Amendments (CLIA)

CLIA stipulates the standards every laboratory must follow during diagnostic procedures, professional qualifications, quality-management systems and the handling of complaints.

Laboratories are inspected regularly to ensure that they are complying with these standards. These are set by the Center for Medicare & Medicaid Service (CMS) or agencies accredited by this center.

Phlebotomists are subjected to these inspections when assigned to perform moderately and highly complex laboratory procedures.

Laboratory procedures are classified into the following categories according to CLIA:

1. **Waived**
   These diagnostic procedures are simple. No training is required. There is little to no risk of error when following the box instructions. Examples include COVID-19 rapid antigen test, home pregnancy test and glucometer testing.

2. **Provider-Performed Microscopy Procedures**
   These procedures require the use of a microscope and are performed by a physician or a dentist in their office. An example is urine microscopy.

3. **Moderate Complexity**
   These procedures require training. They require an understanding of the underlying test principles and knowledge of instrument calibration. Examples include an automated hematology analyzer and a glycohemoglobin analyzer.

4. **High Complexity**
   These procedures utilize complex instrumentation. Interpretation requires higher levels of understanding. The performance of these tests is subjected to proficiency testing. An example is blood culture and antibiotic sensitivity testing.

Chapter 2: Safety Protocols

There are many hazards in the phlebotomist's work environment. Knowledge of these and their associated precautions are important tools you need to use to protect yourself and the patients in your care.

Chain of Infection

Infection-control measures exist in every health care facility. A continuous link between different agents makes up the chain of infection. Consider the following scenarios.

Scenario A. You are asked to perform a newborn screen on a preterm neonate at the nursery. You were recently handling a sputum specimen. You failed to wash your hands and wear gloves during the dermal puncture. The neonate contracts a respiratory infection.

In this situation, the collected sputum specimen (portal of exit) contaminated your unclean hands (reservoir). This served as a vector for transmitting microorganisms (infectious agent) through contact and droplets (mode of transmission) into the neonate's (susceptible host) nose or mouth (portal of entry).

Scenario B. A sick neonate breastfeeds from his mother. She develops a cough. In this case, the neonate (reservoir) transmits the virus or bacteria (infectious agent) from its saliva (portal of exit) through droplets (mode of transmission) to its mother's (susceptible host) nose or mouth (portal of entry).

The chain of infection encompasses six essential components: the source of the infection, the infectious agent itself, the entry points into the host, the transmission method, and the exit points from the host. For a disease to infect a vulnerable host, each of these six elements must be present.

Note from the scenarios that the susceptible host who contracts the disease becomes the new reservoir.

Breaking these links is the aim of infection control. Hazards can be eliminated by strictly implementing hand hygiene and precautions against needlestick injuries.

There are many other potential sources of hazards in the workplace apart from biohazards and sharps. These include chemicals, radioactive material, electrical equipment, fire hazards and physical hazards (i.e., wet floors).

Immunization Requirements for the Health Care Worker

As phlebotomists, you are working closely with potentially infectious material. It is prudent that you be protected from these as much as possible. This is made possible with vaccines.

The following is a list of conditions for which vaccination of health care staff is required:

- Hepatitis B
- Flu (yearly)
- Mumps, measles, rubella
- Varicella
- Diphtheria, tetanus and pertussis

Instead of vaccination, your workplace may require you to have current testing for:

1. Hepatitis B antibody titers
2. Mumps, measles and rubella antibody titers
3. Varicella antibody titers
4. Tuberculin skin tests; if positive, these must be followed up by a chest X-ray

Communicable Diseases

When you have any of these diseases, it is best to avoid contact with others until you are out of the infectious stage:

- Active hepatitis A
- Active tuberculosis
- Bacterial or viral conjunctivitis
- COVID-19 (even if asymptomatic or mild)
- Dysentery
- Flu or influenza
- Herpes zoster
- Infection with lice or scabies
- Measles
- Mumps
- Pertussis
- Streptococcal tonsillitis
- Varicella

Common Pathogens Associated with Antibiotic Resistance Encountered in Health Care Facilities

1. **Methicillin-resistant *Staphylococcus aureus*** causes skin and respiratory infections and systemic sepsis.

2. ***Enterococcus*** attacks susceptible patients with weak immune systems (such as post-transplant patients and HIV/AIDs patients).

3. ***Clostridium difficile*** colonizes the intestines after antibiotic overuse. It is responsible for causing toxic megacolon or pseudomembranous colitis. Clostridia are spore-forming bacilli that do not die off with alcohol-based cleansers. Handwashing with soap and water is recommended when exposed to a patient with this infection.

OSHA Guidelines

The Occupational Safety and Health Administration (OSHA) has implemented guidelines to prevent infections. As discussed, breaking one link in the chain of infection significantly reduces the transmission of diseases.

These guidelines include personal protective equipment (PPE), quarantine and isolation protocols and proper biological waste disposal.

Standard Precautions

Standard precautions are created on the assumption that every person and surface is contaminated and is a potential source of transmissible infection. Therefore, the following is advised:

- Proper hand hygiene
- Correct use of PPE
- Respiratory hygiene or cough/sneeze etiquette
- Having patient-care apparatus
- Environmental awareness
- Proper handling of textiles and laundry

Hand Hygiene

As a certified phlebotomy technician, you work with your hands throughout the day. To protect yourself and patients from transmissible diseases, keep them clean.

Artificial nails are not recommended.

The Centers for Disease Control and Prevention (CDC) recommends washing your hands:

1. Before entering a patient's immediate environment
2. Before performing an aseptic procedure, such as the insertion of an indwelling catheter (even when you will wear gloves)
3. After leaving a patient's bed, room or ward
4. After handling bodily fluids (i.e., blood) or any contaminated surfaces
5. After removing gloves

Using an alcohol-based hand rub is acceptable when your hands are not visibly dirty. Continuously rub your hands until the alcohol dries to maximize its effect. However, alcohol disinfectants are not enough to eradicate *Clostridium* species or spore-forming bacilli.

Handwashing with soap and water is preferred when your hands are visibly dirty.

1. Run your hands under warm water and apply soap to create a lather.
2. Rub both palms in a circular motion.
3. Alternately rub the back of each hand.
4. Clasp your fingers and rub them together.
5. Rub the back of your fingers against each palm.
6. Rub each thumb using the opposite hand.
7. Thoroughly rinse with warm water.

Handwashing should take at least 20 seconds. Dry your hands with a clean paper towel. Reusable towels are avoided in the laboratory, as damp towels create an environment for bacteria to grow.

Ideally, you should not touch the faucet with your hands. If your laboratory does not have automatic or foot pedal faucets, use a paper towel to turn off the tap.

Personal Protective Equipment (PPE)

PPE is designed to limit exposure to infectious material. It must protect the skin, eyes and other possible portals of entry for microorganisms. It usually consists of a gown, facial protection and gloves. In the medical setting, it also includes a biohazard container.

PPEs include the following:

- Mask: Three-layered mask, N95 masks
- Face shield: Optional; required for aerosolizing procedures (i.e., tracheal intubation, airway suctioning, sputum collection)
- Gown: Large enough to cover the entire body and limbs
- Gloves: Size-appropriate

Sequence of Donning

1. Gown: Make sure to adjust the gown properly, tying it securely around your waist and neck.
2. Mask: Secure facial protection by putting on your mask. It must have a snug fit around your nose and mouth—not too tight and not loose. Be sure to apply the mask properly.
3. For masks that require tying, tie them first above and behind your head and then at the neck.
4. For masks that slip on, simply adjust the mask to fit over your nose and mouth with one hand while securing it safely with your other hand.
5. Put on respirators, goggles and face shields, if required.
6. Gloves: Finally, put on your gloves. Make sure that gloves are put over the cuffs of your gown to seal any gaps.

Sequence of PPE Removal

Learning the proper sequence of removing PPE is equally important. The most contaminated items must be removed first. Make sure these do not contact your skin.

The order is gloves first, then goggles or face shields, gown and mask.

Touch only the gloves' and gowns' inside parts and the band or earpiece of the goggles, face shields and masks. Discard each item of PPE as you remove it.

Transmission Precautions

Additional measures need to be taken for highly infectious organisms. Patients may be placed in isolation to prevent transmission when they are highly contagious. Likewise, susceptible or immunocompromised patients may be kept in protective isolation.

Keep up with CDC guidelines. For instance, specialized isolation procedures were established during the Ebola virus outbreak and the COVID-19 pandemic.

Warning signs may be posted on the doors of patient rooms to alert you to transmission-based precautions and the corresponding PPE for these patients.

Airborne precautions protect you from respiratory hazards. Standard precautions are crucial, along with a mask or respirator. Possible airborne infections include adenovirus, mumps, chicken pox, tuberculosis, herpes zoster/shingles and COVID-19.

Droplet precautions, like airborne precautions, are designed to prevent droplets from entering via your skin, eyes or nose after you touch secretions from infected individuals. Standard precautions are crucial, along with a mask or respirator. Use hand hygiene. Possible infections from droplets include adenovirus, mumps, chicken pox, tuberculosis, herpes zoster/shingles and COVID-19.

Contact precautions are designed for organisms that can linger on surfaces. Contact precautions also require standard precautions and proper PPE (including a gown). Possible infections spread from contact include respiratory syncytial virus, diphtheria, influenza, group A *streptococcus*, rhinovirus, scarlet fever and COVID-19.

Always remember to apply standard procedures when handling collected specimens and properly dispose of contaminated items, especially sharps and PPE.

Procedures in Isolation Areas

Before entering **patient rooms with transmission-based precautions**, you must don full PPE. Carry only the equipment necessary for the specified procedure, but do not forget extra tubes. As you leave, you must dispose of everything that entered this environment.

Wipe the outside of the tubes before placing them in a biohazard bag to transport. Take care not to touch the outside of the bag with your contaminated gloves. A double bag may be necessary. Place the tubes in the second bag outside the patient's room.

Before you leave the room, you must remove and discard your PPE. These procedures prevent contaminating the environment outside with airborne pathogens from the room.

Reverse isolation is used for newborns and patients who are immunocompromised or receiving chemotherapy. In these areas, all PPE must be sterile. When you are done with phlebotomy, take all your equipment with you. Remove PPE only after leaving the room. This limits exposure to possible pathogens from outside.

Blood-Borne Pathogens (BBP)

Human immunodeficiency virus (HIV) eventually progresses to immunodeficiency syndrome (AIDS) by attacking CD4 T-lymphocytes. CD4 T-cell titers are used to monitor disease progression. There is no vaccine available for HIV.

Hepatitis B is a virus transmitted through blood and bodily secretions. Infection states vary. They include carrier, acute or chronic infection. The virus attacks the liver cells with symptoms ranging from a flu-like illness to fatal liver carcinoma or cirrhosis. Co-infection with hepatitis D is possible.

A vaccine is available for Hepatitis B. It is provided free of charge to exposed employees, as mandated by OSHA.

Hepatitis C is also an important BBP. No vaccine exists, and infected patients are frequently monitored for HCV viral load.

Needlestick Safety and Prevention Act

Additional protocols enforced by OSHA emphasize innovative engineering solutions to prevent occupational exposures. These include:

- Needle safety devices and appropriate sharps disposal systems
- Properly labeled waste containers
- The mandatory practice of standard precautions
- Prohibition of food and drinks or smoking at workstations
- Prohibition of application of makeup at workstations
- Provision of PPEs to all employees
- Laundry facilities
- Free hepatitis B vaccines
- Ensuring medical attention and follow-up after BBP exposure
- Proper documentation

As a rule of thumb, never recap a needle. OSHA requires needles to be equipped with safety devices.

Once a procedure is complete, dispose of all sharps immediately in biohazard containers resistant to punctures and leaks. These are usually mounted on the walls of patient wards. You can carry a small one in your tray.

When using a syringe attached to a transfer device, throw away the whole assembled unit; do not attempt to disassemble it.

Sharps containers have a marker to designate their capacity. Never fill a container above this mark. Never reach into a container with your bare hands when disposing of sharps.

Postexposure Prophylaxis (PEP)

Report all needlestick incidents and accidental BBP exposures to your supervisor.

For all BBP exposures, OSHA mandates a confidential medical examination to be arranged as soon as possible. When indicated, antibody titers are measured and PEP is given, preferably within 24 hours. Follow-up consultation and testing are provided.

Chemical Hazards

Chemicals are often used in the laboratory, especially for the preparation and processing of samples. These may be caustic or toxic. Always observe labels and follow directions. Never mix any chemicals without training.

Learn to properly use safety showers and eyewashes as a precaution. Immediately wash your skin or eyes in case of chemical contact. You should keep the affected area under running water for 15 to 20 minutes. Seek medical attention.

Biological Waste

All equipment contaminated with bodily fluids or blood must be properly disposed of in bins marked with the biological hazard sign. These are usually color-coded in yellow or red.

Items such as bandages, used gauze, used PPE and alcohol pads belong in the biological waste bin. Urine must be disposed of in the sink in the laboratory.

In case of spills on equipment and surfaces, blood or fluids are first removed with an absorbent material. Do not mop or wipe this off. The area is then disinfected with sodium hypochlorite (1 part diluted in 10 parts water). This should be premixed and prepared in plastic containers in the laboratory.

Types of Biological Waste

- Sharps
  This includes metals or glass with edges that may cut or puncture (examples include needles, surgical blades and broken glass).

- Pathologic or anatomical
  This refers to parts of the human body that have been surgically or accidentally removed (examples include tissues and tumors).

- Infectious
  This refers to soiled tools or supplies contaminated with blood or bodily secretions (bandages, dressings, discarded PPE, masks, etc.).

- Recyclable
  This type of waste may be contaminated and disposable but may still be autoclaved for repeated use, such as plastic syringes (with the needles removed), bottles and catheters.

- Chemical
  This type of waste may include formaldehyde, infected secretions and discarded reagents.

- Pharmaceuticals
  Expired or discarded medicines belong in this category, including cytotoxic drugs, which are potentially hazardous.

Chapter 3: Human Anatomy – The Basics

Anatomical Terms

The phlebotomist and other health care personnel are primarily working with the human body. Every phlebotomist must have a basic knowledge of human anatomy.

First, let us describe how the human body is organized. Each level extends from the previous level, so the whole organism is built up of multiple anatomical systems. These are composed of different organs built from different tissues, which arise as different cells are grouped together.

The building blocks upon which the human body is formed are called **cells**. Each cell has a specific function. For example, each red blood cell functions as a conduit for oxygen. Oftentimes, similar cells group together to perform more complex functions. In this case, they are called **tissues**, of which there are different types. The more common ones are the epithelial, connective, muscular and nervous tissues.

Different types of tissues and their primary functions

- Epithelial tissues cover the lining of the body.
- Connective tissue provides a scaffold of support for the organs.
- Muscles are specialized for movement.
- Nervous tissues are specialized for impulse transmission.

The **organs** are even more complex. A few tissue types compose an organ. For example, the heart comprises cardiac muscle tissue covered by an epithelial lining supported by connective tissues.

The heart and the blood vessels make up the circulatory **system**. A body system is made up of a few organs that perform interrelated functions. Take the urinary system as an example. It eliminates waste and balances the body's pH.

The **kidneys** filter the blood to remove waste and unnecessary ions concentrated in the urine. The urine passes from the kidneys to the **ureters**. The **bladder** stores urine until it is released through the **urethra.**

Body Positions

Body positions are terms that are universally adopted to facilitate communication and discussion among health care workers. They serve as a map of the human body.

The **anatomical position** is the agreed-upon position of the body when relaxed and standing. The head is facing forward while both arms rest at the sides with the palms up.

The **supine** position describes a body lying on its back, while the **prone** position refers to when it is facedown.

Note that anatomical terms indicating direction are usually relative to other body parts.

Directional Terms

DIRECTION	DESCRIPTION	EXAMPLE
Anterior	At the front of or preceding	The frontal lobe is located anterior to the parietal lobes of the brain.
Posterior	Behind	The heart is located posterior to the sternum.
Superior	Above	The adrenal glands are located at the superior poles of the kidneys.
Inferior	Below	The diaphragm is inferior to the lungs.
Proximal	Near the center	The knee is located proximally to the foot.
Distal	Away from the center	The forearm is located distally from the arm.
Lateral	On the side	The ears are on the lateral sides of the head.
Medial	Midline or toward the midline	The median cubital vein is located medial to the cephalic vein.
Ventral	At the front	The palms are ventrally located in the anatomic position.
Dorsal	At the back	The nape is located at the dorsal region of the neck.
Superficial	On the surface	The cornea lies superficially on the eyeball.

Anatomical Planes

The human body is described across different planes. There are four planes.

The frontal plane cuts the body into anterior and posterior sections.
The sagittal plane cuts the body into right and left sections.
The midsagittal plane cuts through vertically into equal right and left sections.
The transverse plane is a cross-section cut horizontally into upper and lower sections.

Body Cavities

Anatomists also describe the position of organs within cavities. There are two major body cavities: the ventral or anterior and the dorsal or posterior. These are subdivided into five minor subcavities.

Within the **ventral cavity** are the thoracic subcavity (enclosing the heart and lungs enclosed in a pleural sheet), abdominal subcavity (enclosing the digestive organs and kidneys) and the pelvic subcavity (enclosing the bladder and internal genitalia).

Within the **dorsal cavity** are the cranial and spinal cavities enclosing the brain and spinal cord, respectively.

Clinicians often describe the abdominal pelvic cavity as existing in quadrants, with the umbilicus midline. This is useful for diagnostic purposes, such that a patient presenting with right upper quadrant pain could have a gallbladder stone or liver disease. The possible source of left lower quadrant pain could be the left ovary or a renal stone.

Integumentary System

This describes the largest organ system of the human body. It is composed of the skin and its associated glands, hair and nails. It is the outermost organ system and thereby acts as a protective barrier and thermal regulator.

The skin prevents microorganisms and chemicals from entering the body's internal environment. It also prevents water from escaping, minimizes water loss and blocks harmful ultraviolet radiation.

The skin insulates the body from the cold and sweats in response to heat. Sweat is produced by the apocrine glands.

Also within the skin are multiple nerve endings specialized in detecting temperature sensations, pain, pressure and deep and light touch.

Layers of the Skin

The **epidermis** is the skin layer exposed to the environment. This is the thinnest layer and is lined by four to five squamous epithelial cells that contain fibrous proteins known as keratin. Keratin forms the external shell and provides waterproofing.

Nails are hard keratin plates that protect the fingers and toes. Hair fiber is made up of keratin as well.

Melanocytes, which produce melanin, are also housed in the epidermis. Melanin is the dark pigment that determines skin color. Exposure to ultraviolet rays induces melanin production. Consequently, the sun-exposed areas of the body are darker.

On the epidermal layer, cells continually die and slough off. This process is called desquamation. This allows the layers to be replaced by younger cells from the deeper layers.

The **dermis** is located right beneath the epidermis. It is thicker and formed from fibrous connective tissue. In contrast, it has a direct blood supply through capillaries and lymphatics. It contains the apocrine and sebaceous glands as well as the hair follicles.

Attaching the dermis to the epidermis are the dermal papillae. These are uneven projections or ridges. The patterns they produce create unique fingerprints and footprints in every individual.

The apocrine glands are located within the dermis and extend up to the epidermis. They regulate body temperature and eliminate waste products from the pores through sweat.

The sebaceous glands produce sebum. This is a type of oil that keeps hair and skin moisturized.

Even deeper than the dermis is the **subcutaneous layer**. It is made up of fat connecting the organs to the skin. It functions as a shock absorber, an energy reserve and insulation.

Common Skin Disorders

Phlebotomists need to recognize certain skin conditions. Areas of the skin afflicted by lesions must be avoided, as they are unsuitable venipuncture sites.

Dermatitis or **contact dermatitis** is an allergic reaction to irritant substances, like soap, cosmetics or certain plants.

Eczema causes an erythematous and pruritic rash in response to an allergen.

Impetigo is from an infection of *Staphylococcus* or *Streptococcus bacteria* or both. It presents as a pus-filled lesion that dries to become a yellowish crust.

Keloid is a type of hypertrophic scar resulting from excess collagen produced during skin healing.

Commonly Ordered Tests for Skin Diseases.

Culture and sensitivity tests from wounds, secretions and lesions for the isolation of pathogenic bacteria and fungi.

Special staining for the identification of pathogens.

Microscopy of skin scrapings fixed in potassium hydroxide to detect fungi.

Punch biopsies to distinguish benign tumors from malignant tumors.

Skeletal System

This is composed of bones, joints and ligaments, which make movement possible in conjunction with the muscles and nerves. The skeletal system provides support and protection. It also stores calcium and phosphorus.

The bone marrow is contained within the long and flat bones and is the site for blood cell formation.

An adult has 206 bones, while a newborn has 300. These bones eventually fuse to form the adult skeletal system.

Common Conditions Affecting the Skeletal System

Joint pain can be either arthralgia or arthritis. **Arthralgia** is due to viral infections or accidents. **Arthritis** involves swelling, erythema and warmth of the overlying skin on the joints, which are absent in arthralgia.

A **fracture** is a break in the bone from accidents or bone abnormalities due to **osteoporosis**, **sarcoma** and other **cancers** involving the bones.

Osteomyelitis is an infection of the bone and its deeper layers, including the marrow. An improper heel puncture traumatizes the bone and can lead to osteomyelitis.

Commonly Ordered Tests Involving the Skeletal System

Synovial fluid, a normally sterile fluid lubricating the joint spaces, can be aspirated to investigate the presence of bacteria and crystals for the diagnosis of joint inflammation or arthritis.

A **wound culture** is performed to identify causative agents in suspected osteomyelitis.

Muscular System

This system coordinates with the skeletal system to provide mobility. It receives signals from the nervous system as well. Tendons connect muscles to bones.

Humans have voluntary and involuntary control over their muscles. Involuntary muscles, such as cardiac muscles, aid in the rhythmic contraction of the heart.

There are three major classifications of muscles in the human body.

Skeletal muscle is a voluntary muscle made up of striated fibers seen on microscopy. It attaches to the bones and makes movement possible.

Smooth muscle is involuntary and nonstriated, thus its name. It lines the walls of the vasculature and internal organs. This muscle allows autonomic functions, like breathing, digestion and micturition, to proceed.

The heart consists of **cardiac muscle**, which contracts rhythmically. Microscopically, it has striae-like skeletal muscle but is not under voluntary control.

Common Conditions Affecting the Muscular System

Atrophy is the loss of muscle bulk from inactivity.

Myalgia is a general medical term to refer to any muscle pain caused by viral infections or accidents.

Poliomyelitis results from a viral infection affecting the nerves which innervate the muscles. It results in a progressive loss of strength and paralysis. Vaccines are available which confer lifelong immunity from this condition.

Commonly Ordered Tests Involving the Musculoskeletal System

TEST	SPECIMEN	DEPARTMENT	CLINICAL CORRELATION
Alkaline phosphatase	Serum or plasma	Chemistry	Multiple myeloma Bone metastasis
Antinuclear antibody	Serum	Immunoserology	Systemic lupus erythematosus, rheumatoid arthritis
Ionized calcium	Serum or plasma; Arterial blood	Chemistry	Ordered when total calcium is abnormal; bone disorders, nephritis
Calcium	Serum or plasma	Chemistry	Hypocalcemia, osteoporosis
Phosphorus	Serum or plasma	Chemistry	Bone disorders, endocrine conditions
Uric acid	Serum or plasma	Chemistry	Renal disorders, gout
Vitamin D	Serum or plasma	Chemistry	Rickets, endocrine disorders
Creatine kinase (CK)	Serum or plasma	Chemistry	Determines the extent of muscular damage
CK isoenzymes MM and MB	Serum	Chemistry	Determines the extent of muscular damage
Lactate dehydrogenase	Serum or plasma	Chemistry	Determines the extent of muscular damage
Magnesium	Serum	Chemistry	Musculoskeletal disorders
Myoglobin	Serum	Chemistry	Determines the extent of muscular damage
Potassium	Serum	Chemistry	Levels are associated with a degree of muscle function

Nervous System

This system primarily functions to recognize and interpret stimuli within a split second to allow time for all the bodily systems to react appropriately (i.e., you instantly remove your hand the moment your fingers touch a hot stove).

The nervous system is composed of neurons. A neuron has a cell body surrounded by branching projections (dendrites) and a single tail (axon). Dendrites receive information through electrical impulses and convey these to the cell body, which sends these out through the axon.

A myelin sheath, produced by Schwann cells, wraps around the axons and dendrites. Myelin allows the impulses to travel more efficiently.

A synapse, the point of impulse transmission, is formed by the communication of an axon with its neighboring dendrites.

The **central nervous system** (CNS) is made up of the brain and spinal cord. The brain is where information is processed, and bodily functions are regulated. The CNS is encased in meningeal layers beneath the skull and the vertebrae. Cerebrospinal fluid flows between these meninges and functions as a shock absorber for the delicate structures within.

Sensory (afferent) neurons receive information from the sensory organs and relay these to the CNS.

Motor (efferent) neurons act in the reverse direction. Impulses originate from the CNS and are relayed either to the muscles to affect contraction or to the glands to affect the release of secretions.

The **peripheral nervous system** (PNS) extends from the CNS to reach all other areas.

The **autonomic nervous system** (ANS) is a function of the PNS. It controls involuntary body functions, such as heart rate, breathing and digestion. Its divisions are assigned as sympathetic or parasympathetic. Responses during a period of stress are regulated by the **sympathetic division**. This allows your pupils to dilate, your heart to beat faster and your digestive functions to momentarily slow down while the vessels dilate to increase blood flow to the brain and muscles. This allows for a quick response to possible threats.

The **parasympathetic division** is dominant during periods of relaxation. It functions opposite to the sympathetic division, lowering the heart rate and regulating normal body activity levels.

Common Conditions Affecting the Nervous System

Amyotrophic lateral sclerosis is a disorder of the CNS that causes progressive musculoskeletal paralysis.

Bell's palsy produces a characteristic paralysis and loss of sensation to one side of the face. It results from compression or swelling of the facial nerve. Its exact cause is unknown, but the triggers include pregnancy, stress, diabetes mellitus and viral infections.

Cerebrovascular accident or **stroke** is due to a blockage of blood flow (from a thrombus or a hemorrhage) to brain areas, resulting in less oxygen supply (or hypoxia). This results in sensory and motor deficits in the face and limbs supplied by the hypoxic area of the brain. The symptoms highly suggestive of stroke are facial asymmetry, slurring of speech and sudden weakness.

Seizures result from abnormal transmission of electrical impulses due to electrolyte imbalances, infections, fever (benign seizures of childhood) or traumatic injury to the brain. Recurring seizures are termed **epilepsy.**

Meningitis refers to swelling of the meninges. **Meningococcal meningitis** from *Neisseria meningitides* is highly contagious.

Parkinson's disease is due to degeneration of the nerves in the substantia nigra of the brain. It causes motor problems, such as slow movements, rigidity and tremors in older people.

The varicella-zoster virus often lies dormant within the peripheral nerves. During periods of immunosuppression, it can reactivate and cause a condition known as **shingles** or **herpes zoster**. This condition is marked by painful blisters along a dermatome, an area supplied by a nerve. This is contagious and causes unvaccinated individuals to develop chicken pox, not shingles.

Commonly Ordered Tests Involving the Nervous System

TEST	SPECIMEN	DEPARTMENT	CLINICAL CORRELATION
CSF cytology	CSF	Hematology	CNS disorders; meningitis
CSF culture and gram stain	CSF	Microbiology	
CSF glucose	CSF	Chemistry	
CSF protein	CSF	Chemistry	
Creatine kinase CK-BB	Serum	Chemistry	Brain damage
Drug screening	Serum	Chemistry	Therapeutic drug monitoring or drug abuse
Lead	Whole blood	Chemistry	Neurologic function
Lithium (Li)	Serum	Chemistry	Drug monitoring for mood disorders

Respiratory System

The primary function of this system is to facilitate gas exchange (or ventilation) among the external environment, the red blood cells and tissues through the process of respiration. Carbon dioxide is exhaled from the lungs into the outer environment in exchange for oxygen.

Internal respiration occurs as gases are exchanged at the level of the red blood cells and internal organs.

These gases circulate through the body through the red blood cells. They bind specifically to a molecule in these cells called **hemoglobin**. Oxygenated blood carries oxyhemoglobin. Only about 20% of carbon dioxide is carried as carboxyhemoglobin. The majority combines with water to form bicarbonate ions circulating through the plasma. As these ions reach the lungs, a chemical reaction allows the carbon dioxide to separate from bicarbonate and bind to the red blood cells. At the alveoli, these diffuse and are released in exhalation.

The levels of circulating oxygen and carbon dioxide are measured from arterial blood as partial pressures. The partial pressure of oxygen should be higher in arterial blood as it functions as the conduit for oxygenated blood.

An analysis of **arterial blood gases** also generates a measurement of body pH. Adequate respiration ensures the proper levels of gases in the body. When respiration is impeded, carbon dioxide is inadequately released, the buildup of which results in a decreased blood pH or respiratory acidosis. The body compensates by increasing the rate of breathing. When this hyperventilation persists, respiratory alkalosis may occur as carbon dioxide is rapidly blown out.

Take note: During venipuncture, a patient may become anxious. Anxiety may produce a sympathetic nervous response observed as increased heart rate and respiration (or hyperventilation).

The respiratory system includes the nose, airway, lungs and alveoli. It is separated into the upper and lower tracts at the level of the carina. Each component performs crucial functions for effective respiration, although ventilation primarily occurs at the alveoli level.

Common Conditions Affecting the Respiratory System

Apnea is a condition when breathing stops involuntarily. This can be observed in premature neonates and resolves spontaneously as the infant matures. **Obstructive sleep apnea** is frequently observed among obese individuals when the weight of their neck compresses their upper respiratory tracts.

Asthma is an inflammation of the small airways triggered by allergens, exercise or smoke, which manifests as shortness of breath and wheezing.

Chronic obstructive pulmonary disease is similar to asthma but develops over time from long-term exposure to tobacco or inhaled irritants.

Cystic fibrosis is a rare genetic condition encountered more in patients of Ashkenazi Jew or Northern European descent. This causes the overproduction of mucous that eventually blocks the bronchioles.

Pertussis causes a characteristic loud "whooping" cough, fever and colds in unvaccinated and susceptible individuals, especially infants under six months of age. Its causative agent is *Bordetella pertussis* bacteria. Immunization of health care staff and those living and working around infants is highly recommended.

Pneumonia refers to an infection resulting in the alveoli filling with fluid. Gas exchange is inadequate; hence the patient appears short of breath and may have oxygen desaturation.

Tuberculosis is a contagious chronic infection due to *Mycobacterium tuberculosis.*

URTI is a commonly encountered abbreviation referring to an infection (either viral or bacterial) involving the organs of the upper respiratory tract. This includes the common cold.

Commonly Ordered Tests for the Respiratory System

TEST	SPECIMEN	DEPARTMENT	CLINICAL ASSOCIATION
Arterial blood gas	Arterial blood	Chemistry	pH balance
Bronchoalveolar lavage	Bronchial washings	Microbiology	Bacterial pneumonia
Cold agglutinin	Serum	Immunoserology	Mycoplasma pneumonia; infectious mononucleosis
Pharyngeal and sputum cultures	Sputum or secretions	Microbiology	Bacterial infection/TB
Pleural fluid analysis	Pleural fluid	Chemistry, microbiology, hematology	Infection, malignancy or organ failure
Sweat chloride test	Sweat	Chemistry	Cystic fibrosis
Complete blood count	Whole blood	Hematology	Infectious diseases, pneumonia

Gastrointestinal System

The gastrointestinal system is responsible for digestive and absorptive functions as well as the elimination of waste products.

The process of digestion begins in the oral cavity. Through mastication, food is mechanically digested by the teeth into particles lubricated by saliva, which pass through the **pharynx** and **esophagus**. They are propelled through this tube by peristalsis. At the level of the **stomach**, the particles are chemically digested by hydrochloric acid secreted by specialized cells. This acidic environment allows for the destruction of pathogenic organisms. *Helicobacter pylori* have the advantage of surviving at this pH level. They are the flagellated bacteria responsible for peptic ulcers and gastric cancers.

The steak and potatoes you recently enjoyed are ground up into a semi-fluid mass called chyme. This reaches the **duodenum** (the first part of the small intestine), where it mixes with the pancreatic juices containing digestive enzymes. The **pancreatic** enzymes catalyze the digestion of specific nutrients, such as amylase for carbohydrates, lipase for fats and chymotrypsin and trypsin for proteins. Additionally, bile, the secretory product of the **gallbladder**, mixes with fat particles and emulsifies it for absorption into the **liver**. Through peristalsis, chyme travels through the length of the small intestine (the duodenum, **jejunum and ileum**) and reaches the colon or the **large intestine**. Here, final absorption occurs and water, minerals and vitamins are absorbed. These are processed in the liver as well. The undigested particles combine to form stool.

Humans do not produce the enzyme called cellulase, which is essential for breaking down cellulose, a compound abundantly found in plants and leafy greens. This unprocessed cellulose forms the majority of our fecal matter and facilitates bowel movements by encouraging the wave-like contractions known as peristalsis, which aid in the easier expulsion of waste.

A low-fiber diet lacking in vegetables contributes to constipation and irritable bowel syndrome.

Lactase, the enzyme which digests lactose (milk sugar), is absent in some people. This deficiency is more common among those of Asian or African descent. **Lactose intolerance** manifests as an upset stomach after eating dairy products.

The main organs of the GI tract include those within the oral cavity (mouth, tongue), thoracic cavity (pharynx and esophagus) and abdominal cavity (stomach, liver, intestines and rectum). The GI tract ends at the anal canal.

Accessory structures include the teeth, salivary glands, pancreas, gallbladder and appendix.

Common Conditions Involving the Gastrointestinal System

Cholecystitis refers to swelling of the gallbladder wall commonly caused by gallbladder or bile duct stones, parasites (Ascaris, liver flukes) or tumors. It may complicate into obstruction of the common bile duct (**cholangitis**), requiring urgent surgical attention.

Cirrhosis refers to the degeneration of hepatic cells from chronic insults to the liver (hepatitis viruses, alcohol, toxins or tumors)

Gastroenteritis is the medical term for diarrhea. It is the inflammation of the gastrointestinal tract resulting in loose stools, abdominal pain, nausea and vomiting. It may be caused by various microorganisms.

Inflammatory bowel disease is an autoimmune condition causing inflammation of the gastrointestinal tract, causing unpredictable episodes of constipation and diarrhea.

Hernia is the abnormal protrusion of a part of an organ through a body cavity that has lost its integrity, such as an inguinal hernia from the protrusion of the mesentery into the inguinal canal.

Pancreatitis causes excruciating abdominal pain from an inflammation of the pancreas. This may be due to excessive alcohol intake, gallbladder stones, cancer or surgical complications.

Peptic or duodenal ulcers are lesions on the epithelium of the stomach due to bacterial infection (*H. pylori*) or excessive acid secretion.

Commonly Ordered Tests for the Gastrointestinal System

TEST	SPECIMEN	DEPARTMENT	ASSOCIATED WITH
Alanine aminotransferase	Serum or plasma	Chemistry	Hepatic function
Albumin	Serum or plasma	Chemistry	Malnutrition; liver function
Alkaline phosphatase	Serum or plasma	Chemistry	Hepatic disorders
Ammonia	Whole blood	Chemistry	Severe hepatic disorders
Amylase	Serum or plasma	Chemistry	Pancreatitis
Aspartate aminotransferase	Serum or plasma	Chemistry	Hepatic disorders
Bilirubin	Serum or plasma	Chemistry	Hepatic disorders
Carcinoembryonic antigen (CEA)	Serum	Chemistry	Carcinoma detection and monitoring
Complete blood count	Whole blood	Hematology	Infections
Gamma-glutamyl transferase (GGT)	Serum	Chemistry	Early hepatic disorders
Gastrin	Serum	Chemistry	Gastric malignancy
Hepatitis A, B and C immunoassays	Serum	Immunoserology	Hepatitis A, B and C screening
Lactate dehydrogenase	Serum or plasma	Chemistry	Hepatic disorders
Lipase	Serum or plasma	Chemistry	Pancreatitis
Occult blood	Stool	Microscopy	Gastrointestinal bleeding or colorectal cancers
Ova and parasites (O & P)	Stool	Microscopy	Parasitic infection
Stool culture	Stool	Microscopy	Bacterial pathogens
Total protein (TP)	Serum	Chemistry	Hepatic disorders

Urinary System

The urinary system's primary functions are eliminating water-soluble byproducts of metabolism and balancing the body's pH, electrolytes and water. It is composed of the bladder, kidneys, ureters and urethra.

The **kidneys** are a pair of bean-shaped structures containing over a million nephrons each. They act as a blood filtration and ion reabsorption system. As blood leaves the **nephrons**, it circulates through a bundle of capillaries—the **glomerulus**, which acts as a sieve. This removes smaller substances while retaining larger ones, such as red cells and proteins. Through the long tubules of the nephrons, selective filtration occurs. Water, glucose, hydrogen, bicarbonate ions and electrolytes may be reabsorbed to maintain homeostasis. The substances discarded by the nephrons form urine. This passes from each kidney to the paired ureters. It is stored in the bladder until the detrusor muscles contract to allow for **micturition** (urination).

The volume of urine correlates with the hydration status. Typically, about one liter of urine is formed every day. Certain patients, especially those requiring intensive care, need to have their fluid intake and urine output recorded regularly, as often as every hour, to monitor the status of their kidneys or prevent dehydration.

Kidney function is estimated through the **glomerular filtration rate**, which should be 90 to 120 $ml/min/1.73m^2$. This means all the blood travels through the kidney's filtration system about 40 times a day.

Creatinine is a substance that is excreted in the urine. It is neither secreted nor reabsorbed in the nephrons. It is formed after muscle metabolism and is normally found in only small amounts in the blood. This makes it an excellent estimate of the glomerular filtration rate. Increased blood creatinine correlates with a decreased GFR. GFR is calculated through a formula factoring the patient's weight, age, gender and creatinine. This makes creatinine an important test for kidney function.

The kidneys also have endocrine functions. They produce **renin**, which is involved in blood pressure regulation, and **erythropoietin**, which signals the bone marrow to produce red blood cells. The kidneys are also responsible for converting exogenous vitamin D (from the sun or diet) into its active bioavailable form.

Common Conditions Involving the Urinary System

Cystitis refers to an inflamed urinary bladder, probably from a bacterial infection or a **urinary tract infection**, whereas **pyelonephritis** refers to an inflamed renal pelvis.

Nephrolithiasis is the medical term for a kidney stone. These form when there is too much of certain substances, such as uric acid or calcium, in the blood, which exceeds the kidneys' filtering capacity. Urine cannot dilute these substances adequately. Over time, they clump together and form hard deposits along the urinary tract. Kidney stones may be very painful to pass and sometimes block urine flow. This condition may require surgical intervention.

Renal failure refers to the complete loss of kidney function in one or both kidneys. Often, it is detected when both have failed. It may progress as **uremia**, wherein blood contains too much urea and metabolic wastes. Uremia and severe renal failure indicate the need for hemodialysis.

Commonly Ordered Tests for the Urinary System

TEST	SPECIMEN	DEPARTMENT	ASSOCIATED WITH
Creatinine	Serum or plasma	Chemistry	Renal function
Albumin	Serum or plasma	Chemistry	Renal disorders
Ammonia	Whole blood	Chemistry	Renal function
Blood urea nitrogen	Serum or plasma	Chemistry	Renal function; increase in uremia
Electrolytes	Serum or plasma	Chemistry	Fluid balance
Osmolality	Serum	Chemistry	Fluid and electrolyte balance
Total protein	Serum	Chemistry	Renal disorders
Uric acid	Serum	Chemistry	Renal function
Urinalysis	Urine	Microscopy	Renal or metabolic disorders
Urine culture and sensitivity	Urine	Microbiology	Bacterial infection

Endocrine System

The endocrine system regulates metabolism, sleep, stress and reproduction through hormones. It closely coordinates with the nervous system.

The **hypothalamus** is responsible for producing and secreting releasing hormones. These signal the **anterior pituitary gland** to release a corresponding stimulating hormone. These, in turn, signal the endocrine organs to secrete their hormones. The body utilizes a feedback system to increase or decrease the levels of circulating hormones.

For example, thyrotropin-releasing hormones from the hypothalamus signal the anterior pituitary glands to release thyroid-stimulating hormones. These, in turn, signal the thyroid glands to secrete thyroid hormones. Thyroid hormones bind with specialized receptors on different organs and regulate multiple functions. The table below lists the different hormones and their functions.

ENDOCRINE ORGAN	HORMONE	FUNCTIONS
Anterior pituitary gland	Thyroid-stimulating hormone	Signals the release of thyroxine and triiodothyronine (thyroid hormones)
	Adrenocorticotropic hormone	Signals the adrenal glands to release cortisol
	Growth hormone	Responsible for bone development
	Follicle-stimulating hormone	Regulates reproductive functions but stimulates the growth of ovarian follicles in women and the development of male spermatozoa
	Luteinizing hormone	Regulates reproductive functions but stimulates ovulation in women and production of testosterone in men
	Prolactin	Signals lactation and breast development
	Melanocyte-stimulating hormone	Controls the deposition of melanin in the skin
Posterior pituitary gland	Antidiuretic hormone	Regulates the kidneys to reabsorb water and influences hydration
	Oxytocin	In females, it stimulates the uterus to contract and the mammary glands to secrete milk (or lactate).
Thyroid gland	Thyroxine and triiodothyronine	Regulates metabolic functions and influences energy production

	Calcitonin	Regulates calcium and phosphate balance; decreases reabsorption of these minerals from the bones
Parathyroid gland	Parathyroid hormones	Opposes the action of calcitonin; regulates calcium and phosphate balance and increases reabsorption of these minerals from the bones
Adrenocortical gland	Aldosterone	Responsible for sodium and potassium regulation; affects blood pressure
	Cortisol	Increases in response to stress; responsible for metabolic functions and has anti-inflammatory properties
Adrenal medullary gland	Epinephrine and norepinephrine	Increases in response to stress; increases heart rate and activity; produces vasoconstriction and increased blood pressure
	Estrogen and androgens	Responsible for secondary sexual development
Pancreas	Glucagon	Catabolizes glycogen to release glucose into the bloodstream to increase blood sugar
	Insulin	Anabolic hormone; stores glucose in the blood cells; decreases blood sugar levels
Ovaries	Progesterone	Regulates functions of the female reproductive system; responsible for maintenance of pregnancy
	Estrogen	Responsible for female secondary sexual development
Testes	Testosterone	Stimulates the maturation of sperm cells; responsible for male secondary sexual development
Thymus	Thymosin	Stimulates the maturation of T cells; responsible for developing the immune system; atrophies in adults
Pineal gland	Melatonin	Regulates the circadian rhythm; stimulated by darkness and allows sleep to occur

Common Conditions Affecting the Endocrine System

Acromegaly is a condition resulting from the excessive secretion of growth hormones, leading to a progressive and noticeable enlargement of extremities like hands and feet. Additionally, it is associated with the development of distinctive, coarse features on the face.

Diabetes insipidus is caused by inadequate levels of antidiuretic hormones. Water is not adequately reabsorbed by the kidneys. It manifests as excess thirst and excess urination.

Dwarfism is due to the lack of growth hormones during development. This results in a short stature but well-proportioned limbs.

Congenital hypothyroidism is observed in infants with impaired thyroid function due to a genetic disorder or maternal iodine deficiency. If left undetected, it may lead to growth and intellectual impairment.

Goiter refers to an enlarged thyroid gland.

Graves' disease refers to increased cellular metabolism from hyperthyroidism.

Hyperparathyroidism results from excess parathyroid hormone. This causes hypercalcemia due to excessive bone resorption. It affects the bones (pain, fractures) and causes kidney stones, lethargy, depression and abdominal upset.

Diabetes mellitus results from increased blood sugar due to insulin deficiency or the inability of cell membrane receptors to recognize insulin.

Addison's disease is a disorder of the adrenal glands and is also known as **adrenal insufficiency**. The glands do not secrete sufficient cortisol and aldosterone. This results in fatigue and body pain.

Cushing's disease is from the excessive secretion of adrenocorticotropic hormone, which results in excessive cortisol levels. This may be due to a pituitary or adrenal gland tumor.

Commonly Ordered Tests for the Endocrine System

TEST	SPECIMEN	DEPARTMENT	CLINICAL CORRELATION
Adrenocorticotropic hormone (ACTH)	Whole blood	Chemistry	Pituitary or adrenal tumors
Aldosterone	Serum	Chemistry	Addison's disease
Antidiuretic hormone (ADH)	Whole blood	Chemistry	Diabetes insipidus
Calcium (Ca)	Serum or plasma	Chemistry	Hyperparathyroidism
Cortisol	Serum	Chemistry	Cushing's disease
Glucose	Serum or plasma	Chemistry	Hypoglycemia, diabetes mellitus
Glycosylated hemoglobin	Serum or plasma	Chemistry	Diabetes mellitus
Growth hormone (GH)	Serum or plasma	Chemistry	Acromegaly
Insulin level	Serum	Chemistry	Glucose metabolism and pancreatic function
Parathyroid hormone (PTH)	Whole blood	Chemistry	Hyperparathyroidism or hypoparathyroidism
Testosterone	Serum	Chemistry	Polycystic ovarian syndrome
Thyroid function (T3, T4, TSH) studies	Serum	Chemistry	Hypothyroidism or hyperthyroidism

Reproductive System

The organs of this system are designed for copulation and reproduction. The male and female bodies have different yet complementary organs. The vital functions of this system are to produce gametes and, in women, to sustain a favorable environment for the development of the embryo.

The Female Reproductive Anatomy

The ovaries contain **ova**. An ovum holds half of the human genetic material. It is produced from immature ovarian follicles. This begins during menarche (onset of a girl's first menstruation) and ends during menopause.

An ovum is released during ovulation and travels through the **fallopian tubes**, where it awaits spermatozoa to fertilize it. A fertilized ovum becomes the **embryo**. It is implanted into the uterus. Here, it undergoes multiple cell divisions and forms the fetus. The fetus is nourished within the placenta. It receives nutrients from the mother through the umbilical vessels.

The hormone **progesterone**, together with **human beta chorionic gonadotropin** (detected in serum and urine pregnancy test kits), is increased at this time to help maintain the pregnancy. After 40 weeks, the fetus is delivered as a neonate.

If no spermatozoa are received after ovulation, the ovum atrophies and the uterine lining sheds in the process called menstruation. It then prepares for the next cycle.

The Male Reproductive Anatomy

The **testes** lie within the scrotal sac. They are responsible for producing **testosterone**. The male gametes are called **spermatozoa**. They are stored in the **epididymis** and mature there. They then travel the length of the **vas deferens** and get propelled to the **ejaculatory duct**. Here spermatozoa are admixed with fluids and nutrients from the **seminal vesicles** and **prostate gland** and become **semen**. During ejaculation, semen is propelled through the **penile urethra**. At this point, it carries additional fluids from the **bulbourethral glands** to aid in its survival in the female reproductive tract.

Common Conditions Affecting the Reproductive System

Sexually transmitted diseases cause inflammation or lesions in the genital organs. Common bacteria and their corresponding disease include:

- *Chlamydia trachomatis* (chlamydia)
- *Trichomonas vaginalis* (trichomoniasis)
- Herpes simplex virus (herpes genitalis)
- *Treponema pallidum* (syphilis)
- *Neisseria gonorrhea* (gonorrhea)

Pelvic inflammatory disease is due to an infection that affects the organs of reproduction and may cause infertility or septicemia.

Endometriosis results from abnormal implantation of endometrial tissue outside the uterus. This may result in abnormal uterine bleeding.

Commonly Ordered Tests Involving the Reproductive System

TEST	SPECIMEN	DEPARTMENT	CLINICAL CORRELATION
Amniocentesis	Amniotic fluid		Maturity of the fetus; congenital defects
Chorionic villus sampling	Chorionic villus		Congenital defects; Down syndrome
Estradiol, estriol and estrogen	Serum	Chemistry	Function of the ovaries or placenta
Genital culture	Genital secretions swabs		Sexually transmitted diseases
Human chorionic gonadotropin	Serum or plasma	Chemistry	Pregnancy
Papanicolaou smear	Cervical swab		Cervical cancer
Prostate-specific antigen	Serum	Chemistry	Prostate cancer
Fluorescent treponemal antibody-absorption	Serum	Immunoserology	Treponema pallidum
Rapid plasma reagin	Serum	Immunoserology	Treponema pallidum
Venereal disease research laboratory	Serum	Immunoserology	Treponema pallidum
Rubella titer	Serum	Immunoserology	Rubella infection or immunity
Semen analysis	Semen		Fertility studies
Testosterone	Serum	Chemistry	Male characteristic, polycystic ovarian syndrome
Toxoplasma antibody screening			Toxoplasma infection

Circulatory System

This system is composed of a series of pumps (the heart and its chambers) and tubes (the blood vessels) through which blood circulates. The main role of the blood is to transport oxygen and nutrients while removing waste.

The Vasculature

These are the blood vessels that act as highways for blood cells. The **arteries** carry oxygen-rich blood, while the **veins** carry oxygen-poor blood. **Capillary** beds in the tissues are suitable for exchanging nutrients, wastes and gases.

The histologic structure of the blood vessels is designed to facilitate its functions. The walls are made up of three layers, starting from the outermost to the innermost: tunica adventitia, made up of connective tissue; tunica media, which is both muscular and elastic; and tunica intima, which is lined by endothelium.

The Arteries

The **arteries** are larger and thicker blood vessels. Their structure is necessary to counter the high pressures of the contracting heart ventricles. This allows the arteries to propel oxygenated blood from the heart into the smaller blood vessels. They branch into smaller **arterioles**, which communicate with the capillaries. This is where gas exchange occurs. For this purpose, arterioles are also lined with smooth muscles to maintain a pulsating pressure to distribute blood into these smaller structures.

Some common examples of arteries encountered in the health care setting are:

- **Aorta**: This is the largest artery, which stems directly from the heart.
- **Radial arteries**: These run along the lateral area of each wrist. Their pulse is felt on the ventral surface right below the thumb.
- **Carotid arteries**: These are large arteries supplying blood to the brain. They branch from the aorta. The pulse is felt on either side of the neck. It is the most common site to identify a pulse during emergencies.
- **Brachial arteries**: These run along the antecubital fossa. Their pulsations are felt along the lower edge of the elbow crease. These arteries are compressed by a sphygmomanometer or blood pressure cuff to determine blood pressure.
- **Femoral arteries**: These are located at the inguinal canal. This is one of the sites for arterial blood collection.

The Veins

The **veins** are thinner. Deoxygenated blood courses through them. It carries carbon dioxide and waste back to the heart. The tunica media of these vessels contains less elastic tissue, as it is not subjected to higher pressure. Blood is propelled through the veins by the contraction of the surrounding muscles. It is also equipped with valves to prevent blood from backing up. The veins in the lower limbs contain many valves, as they must overcome gravity to return blood to the heart.

Most phlebotomy work involves the manipulation of veins. The term *venipuncture* refers to the puncturing of veins to draw out blood. The choice veins for venipuncture are superficial and can be palpated in the **antecubital fossa of the forearm**. These veins are called the **median cubital**, **cephalic** and **basilic**. These all branch off the dorsal venous plexus of the hands and drain into the axillary vein.

The other important veins encountered in the health care setting include:

- **Superior vena cava**: This is a large vein that drains the vessels above the heart.
- **Inferior vena cava**: This drains blood from the vessels below the heart.
- **Great saphenous vein**: This is in the leg and is the longest vein in the body.
- **Pulmonary vein**: This is notable, as it is the only vein that does not carry deoxygenated blood.

The Capillaries

Capillaries are unique blood vessels composed of a single layer of endothelial cells, without the typical tunica media and adventitia found in other vessels. This streamlined structure allows them to be permeable to gases like oxygen and carbon dioxide, along with other metabolic waste products. Importantly, capillaries serve as the site where oxygen-rich and oxygen-poor blood intermingle.

Common Conditions Affecting the Vasculature

Aneurysm is the outpouching of a blood vessel wall layer due to weakness. It is a serious condition, as it may progress, increase in size or burst, leading to a hemorrhage. Dangerous sites of aneurysm are the abdominal aorta and the brain.

Arteriosclerosis refers to a hardened or sclerotic artery wall. This increases the risk of a cerebrovascular accident or aneurysm.

Atherosclerosis refers to the narrowing of the blood vessel lumen from an accumulation of fats and trapped cells. These form into a clot and may break away suddenly in the form of emboli. An **embolism** occurs when an emboli lodges into a smaller vessel and obstructs blood flow, causing ischemia. Emboli are often responsible for myocardial infarction, pulmonary embolism and cerebrovascular accidents.

Phlebitis is a condition that phlebotomists can inflict if they are not being careful. This refers to pain and swelling of the vein. An indwelling IV cannula can also be the culprit in this condition.

Thrombosis refers to a blood clot obstructing blood flow through the vessels.

The Heart

This is the muscular pump within the thorax. It is protected by the sternum and the intercostal bones within the rib cage. It is lined by a layer of the pericardium. It is located between the right and left lungs and slightly on the left.

The epicardium is the outermost layer of the heart. It is composed of connective tissue, mesothelium and adipose cells. The middle layer is muscular, and it is aptly called the myocardium. A layer of epithelium, comprising the endocardium, lines the inner chambers.

The Chambers of the Heart

The cavities in the heart are organized into four chambers. There are two **atria** and two **ventricles**. A septum separates them into the right and left halves.

Cardiac Valves

Like the valves in the veins, the heart valves direct blood unidirectionally. They are located at the openings of the ventricles.

The **aortic** and **pulmonary** valves are semilunar, while the **mitral (bicuspid)** and **tricuspid** valves have cusps.

The Pathway of Blood

From both the vena cava and the carotid sinus, deoxygenated blood enters the **right atrium**. After passing through the **tricuspid valve**, it empties into the **right ventricle**. This pumps the blood through the **pulmonary valves**. Blood enters the pulmonary arteries and reaches the pulmonary circulation. Here, it exchanges its carbon dioxide for oxygen.

Oxygenated blood then returns through the **pulmonary veins** and enters the heart at the **left atrium**. It passes the **mitral valves** on its way to the left ventricle. The next contraction pushes the now oxygen-rich blood through the **aortic valves** back to the systemic circulation through the **aorta**.

Cardiac Circulation

The heart also requires oxygen to perform its functions adequately. It is nourished by its complex vascular system. The right and left coronary arteries branch off from the aorta into smaller arteries to reach the coronary capillaries and supply each atrium and ventricle of the heart. Oxygen-poor blood then enters the heart through the coronary sinus.

The Cardiac Cycle

The heart contracts rhythmically. This is known as the **cardiac cycle.** With each contraction or systole, blood is pumped into the lungs and the aorta. With each relaxation or diastole, blood fills the chambers of the heart.

The cardiac muscle contracts autonomously. It is controlled by electrical impulses originating from the SA node (the native pacemaker). It travels through the AV node, AV bundles and bundle branches (right and left) until reaching the Purkinje fibers at the ventricles. This process initiates cardiac contraction.

An **electrocardiogram** (commonly referred to as an ECG) measures the cardiac cycle. Electrodes are placed on all four limbs. Six electrodes are arranged on the chest. These record the heart's electrical activity. An ECG gives information on the time for one heartbeat or cardiac cycle to complete, as well as the regularity of the heart's rhythm. Clinicians determine the timing of each atrial and ventricular systole and diastole by understanding the relationship of the waves and crests on the ECG tracing. An ECG is indispensable for the diagnosis of heart conditions.

The Pulse

The heart typically beats 60 to 90 times per minute. When you are feeling someone's pulse, you are feeling the rhythmic waves traveling through the arteries from the pumping heart. Common areas to locate the pulse are the neck (carotid artery), the anterior elbow crease (brachial artery) and the wrist (radial artery).

When checking the pulse rate in your patients, it is easier to locate the radial artery pulse. Press the pads of your index and middle fingers over the radius. Record the heart rate. This is done by counting the number of beats for half a minute, then multiplying it by two. Check for rhythm. If it is irregular, count the rate for a full minute. Assess the strength of the pulse. For example, the pulse rate is fully reported as "80 bpm, regular, bounding."

Bradycardia refers to a pulse rate below 60 bpm, while **tachycardia** is a rate above 100 bpm.

Blood Pressure Determination

Blood pressure determines the pressure on the blood vessel walls during systole and diastole. It is measured in millimeters of mercury and reported as two numbers. The one above is the systole, while the one below is the diastole. This is normally 120/80 mmHg for adults.

A **sphygmomanometer** is an apparatus used to measure BP. An inflatable cuff is placed over the upper arm, two inches over the elbow crease, while a stethoscope is positioned at the antecubital fossa over the brachial artery. As the cuff inflates, the blood vessel is constricted. Deflating the cuff slowly allows the examiner to determine the pressure (over the pressure gauge) by which the first heart sound is heard. This is recorded as systolic BP. The cuff is deflated further until the sounds disappear. This is recorded as diastolic BP.

Common Conditions Affecting the Heart

Angina pectoris refers to pain over the chest from ischemia to the heart. It is often due to atherosclerosis or emboli in the coronary arteries.

Endocarditis is the inflammation of the endocardium, often due to bacteria.

Myocardial infarction is commonly referred to as a heart attack. This is from a severe lack of oxygen to an area of the heart, leading to necrosis.

Pericarditis is the inflammation of the pericardium from microorganisms or trauma.

Blood

On average, the human adult has about five to six liters of blood. Blood is a suspension of cells over a liquid known as plasma.

Blood is about 55% **plasma**. When separated, it is clear and straw-colored. It is mostly water with some dissolved substances, such as proteins, vitamins, hormones and wastes.

The rest are **formed elements.** These are the erythrocytes (red blood cells), leukocytes (white blood cells) and thrombocytes (platelets).

An erythrocyte lives for up to 120 days, after which it is sequestered in the spleen. The iron and heme it carries are recycled for new cells.

Blood Group Systems

The erythrocytes can be coated with antigens. These determine a person's blood type. It can either be A, B or AB, depending on which antigen is present. The O blood type contains no antigens.

The corresponding antibodies for antigens absent on an erythrocyte are found in the plasma. Therefore, people with type A blood will develop a transfusion reaction after receiving type B or AB. Their plasma contains anti-B antibodies that attack the B antigen on the donated blood cells.

However, these people can receive type O blood since it contains no antigens. Type O is known as the universal donor blood type.

Type AB is considered the universal receiver. It has no anti-A or anti-B antibodies.

Note to phlebotomists: Always properly identify each patient to avoid a possibly fatal transfusion reaction.

Rh Factor

The **D antigen** may be present or absent on the erythrocytes. This is also known as the **Rh factor**. It is reported as positive or negative. This forms eight common blood groups.

- A positive
- A negative
- B positive
- B negative
- O positive
- O negative
- AB positive
- AB negative

Unlike the blood type antigens, Rh-negative individuals do not have naturally occurring antibodies to the Rh factor. They must first encounter Rh-positive blood through transfusion or pregnancy, after which their plasma retains the memory in the form of anti-D antibodies.

A second transfusion of Rh-positive blood will result in a transfusion reaction. In pregnancy, this is known as **hemolytic disease of the newborn.**

The White Blood Cells

These cells, also known as **leukocytes,** protect the body from harmful microorganisms. They are normally present in the blood at a level of 4,500 to 11,000/microliter. A differential count identifies five different forms of leukocytes and reports the percentage of each.

Neutrophils are the most abundant. They average 40% to 60% of the total leukocytes. They are the first-line defense against pathogens as they phagocytose these. These cells proliferate in response to bacterial infections.

Lymphocytes comprise 20% to 40%. They confer immunity through the B and T cells. They proliferate in response to viral infections.

Monocytes are large leukocytes that are normally found at 3% to 8%. They are powerful phagocytes. When found in the tissues, they go by different names—alveolar macrophages in the lungs, osteoclasts in the bone, microglia in the CNS and Kupffer cell in the liver. Monocytes proliferate in the presence of chronic intracellular infections and tuberculosis.

Eosinophils form only 1% to 3%, but they have unique responsibilities. They detoxify foreign proteins and proliferate in response to allergens and parasites.

Basophils are even fewer and sometimes absent at 0% to 1%. They are responsible for histamine response during inflammatory processes. They also contain granules of heparin to prevent blood clots.

The Platelets

These are also known as **thrombocytes**. They are irregular disks that chip off a much larger cell called the **megakaryocyte.** They remain in the blood for about 9 to 12 days and number, on average, at about 140,000/microliter to 440,000/microliter. They are necessary for the coagulation process.

Common Conditions Affecting the Blood

Anemia refers to low levels of hemoglobin in the blood.

Leukemia is a type of cancer resulting in an excessive increase in certain leukocytes.

Leukocytosis refers to an increase in the number of white blood cells, such as during infections.

Leukopenia is the decrease in the number of white blood cells. This is a complication of chemotherapy or radiation treatment.

Polycythemia refers to the abnormal increase in the levels of erythrocytes or hematocrit.

Thrombocytopenia refers to low levels of platelets (thrombocytes). This may interfere with wound healing. When the levels are very low, spontaneous bleeding can occur.

Thrombocytosis refers to an increased level of platelets.

Coagulation and Hemostasis

Hemostasis refers to the formation of blood clots in response to a blood vessel injury. This prevents blood from leaking out. When the injury has been repaired, it signals factors to lyse the clot. These processes involve a complex mechanism involving platelets and clotting factors, which may be described in four stages.

Primary Hemostasis

Immediately after an injury, the vasculature constricts to prevent blood from leaking out. Platelets aggregate and clump (aggregation). They adhere to the injured area (adhesion) as a temporary plug.

A platelet count is ordered to determine whether the patient adequately forms a platelet plug during this stage of hemostasis.

Secondary Hemostasis or the Coagulation Cascade

At this point, fibrin strands are formed into a fibrin clot, which strengthens the platelet plug. The coagulation cascade can be initiated by either of two pathways.

The **extrinsic pathway** is stimulated after external tissue damage by the tissue factor, while the **intrinsic pathway** becomes activated by glass (in vitro) or endothelial collagen (in vivo).

This stage of hemostasis is evaluated by coagulation tests. The **prothrombin time** can estimate the function of the extrinsic pathway and is useful in monitoring the response to warfarin therapy. The **activated partial thromboplastin time (APTT)** can estimate the function of the intrinsic pathway.

These pathways meet at the common pathway and continue the cascade of clotting factors.

Fibrin Clot

The cascade ends after factor XIII is activated. At this point, the fibrin clot is stabilized and the clot retracts or tightens.

Evaluation of this stage is possible by measuring the **thrombin time** or the amounts of **fibrinogen**.

Clot Lysis

Once the blood vessel has healed from the initial insult, the fibrin clot is broken down into **fibrin degradation products** during fibrinolysis. Therefore, measurement of fibrin degradation products and its protein fragment, **D-dimer**, can provide an estimate of the extent of fibrinolysis.

Common Conditions Involving the Coagulation Pathways

Deep vein thrombosis occurs when a clot forms deep within the vein, causing pain, inflammation and enlargement of the veins in the affected area.

Disseminated intravascular coagulation happens when pathogens, such as during sepsis, trigger the coagulation system to activate all over the body. This consumes a lot of the clotting factors and often complicates spontaneous bleeding.

Hemophilia is an inherited condition from the lack of factor VIII or IX. This presents in early childhood as excess bleeding or easy bruising from the inadequate function of hemostasis.

Chapter 4: Routine Blood Collection Materials

Professional phlebotomists keep their workstations organized and ensure the materials are ready for the next venipuncture procedure.

Routine equipment includes evacuated tube holders, needles, different-sized syringes, winged collection sets, collection tubes tourniquets, antiseptic skin preparation solutions (povidone-iodine swabs, chlorhexidine swabs, 70% alcohol swabs), gloves, gauze pads, slides, markers and pencil, transfer devices and a sharps disposal container. An alcohol-based hand gel should also be carried or made readily accessible.

The phlebotomist is often called to collect blood from a patient's ward. A phlebotomy tray is designed to carry all the needed equipment. It should be refilled and sanitized at least once a week. This prevents errors and inconveniences when collecting blood.

Evacuated Tube System

This is the most common method of venipuncture utilizing an evacuated tube or ETS. It has a double-pointed (multisample) needle. The unsheathed end punctures the vein, while another end (sheathed in a holder) punctures a collection tube. This system relies on a predetermined vacuum that automatically fills each evacuated tube. This eliminates manual specimen transfer, thereby decreasing the risk of exposure to biological hazards. It also ensures the correct blood-to-additive ratio to avoid incorrect test results.

Needles

Needles may be multisample, hypodermic or part of a winged set. They are usually described by gauge and length. Needles are packaged individually and come with a sterile shield and color-coded hub for easy identification.

The phlebotomist chooses the right needle for venipuncture to ensure patient comfort while minimizing the risk of complications.

A needle gauge indicates the size of its diameter. It can range from 16 to 25. A lower number indicates a thicker needle. A 21-gauge needle is thinner than a 16-gauge needle.

A 21-gauge is the standard size of needle for most adults. Larger gauges are used for children and adults with smaller veins.

A 25-gauge needle is avoided for venipuncture. The narrow diameter can cause hemolysis. This may cause potassium and magnesium to leak out of the cells and falsely increase serum determinations. It also causes a false decrease in red cell count, hematocrit and APTT values.

The 20-gauge needle is also avoided. Patients on blood thinners may experience bleeding and hematomas after the procedure from the larger injury on the vein.

The length of the hypodermic needles is usually an inch to an inch and a half, while winged collection needles are 0.5 to 0.75 inches.

The structure of a needle varies when it is hypodermic, multisample or part of a winged collection set. All needles have a hub, shaft, bevel and point.

It is important to look at your needle before you use it. Look for defects, like an absent bevel or breaks. If a needle is defective, discard it in the sharps container. Never recap a needle, used or unused.

Needle Holder

Double-pointed needles are attached to a needle holder. This is a clear, firm plastic and may come with a safety device. They are available in various types to fit collection tubes of varying sizes. These must fit securely.

The ETS mainly uses this system. As one point of the needle inserts into the vein, blood is vacuumed through the other point into the evacuated tubes. This vacuum is created by puncturing the rubber stopper of the collecting tube with a rubber-sheathed needle. Each evacuated tube comes with a predetermined vacuum.

When the tubes have filled, slightly twist them to remove them. When collecting multiple tubes, secure the needle first by firmly grasping the holder through its flanges. This holds the needle in the vein and avoids puncturing it.

Needle Safety Features

The Needlestick Prevention and Safety Act mandates that every needle has a safety feature. This may be a device that blunts, shields or retracts the needle after use. After performing venipuncture, you should activate the safety device.

Blood Collection Tubes

Blood collection tubes or **evacuated tubes** are specialized containers used to collect and transport blood samples. There are varying sizes that can collect from 1.8 up to 15 milliliters of blood. Each tube is sterile and designed for specific purposes. It may or may not contain an additive. It may be made of glass or plastic. Glass tubes are generally avoided since these may break and increase the risk of BBP exposure.

The phlebotomist selects the appropriate tube based on the patient's age and veins, the tests being ordered and the amount of blood required.

Tubes have a thick rubber stopper, which is thinner in the center for puncturing. It comes with a color-coded shield to prevent splatters. The colors vary by the type of additives coated in the tube. The colors are generally universal, with slight variations per manufacturer.

Removal of tube stoppers should be avoided. They cause aerosols and may spread BBPs. When necessary, open the tube by covering the stopper with a gauze pad and loosening it slowly, directed away from you.

Evacuated tubes in the ETS fill automatically to a predetermined level. Tubes that fill partially usually have a white ring on the cap.

Each tube is labeled with its additives, volume and expiration date.

Tubes that have already lost their vacuum may cause a failed collection.

Factors that can cause a tube to lose its vacuum are:

- Manufacturer error
- Expired tubes
- Dropped tubes
- Opened or punctured tubes
- Improperly stored tubes
- Improper venipuncture technique (i.e., the tube is advanced too soon; the bevel is dislodged accidentally)

Blood Collection Tube Additives

A test may require either whole blood or only serum or plasma. Some test determinants may need certain chemicals to act as stabilizers, preservatives or anticoagulants. Tubes contain these chemicals, which are called **additives**.

Anticoagulants may be required for tests using whole blood to prevent coagulation, which interferes with the reading of the results. These chemicals prevent the formation of a blood clot by binding calcium (**ethylenediaminetetraacetic acid**) or inhibiting thrombin (**heparin**). These tubes must be inverted an appropriate number of times to properly mix and prevent microclots. Do not shake. Shaking may cause hemolysis. The formation of air bubbles through the tube while inverting ensures adequate mixing.

Some tubes use a powdered form of anticoagulants. When using these, tap the tube gently to loosen the particles and ensure proper mixing.

Do not transfer blood from an additive-containing tube into another tube with other additives. This produces contamination and incorrect test results.

A color-coding system helps identify which tubes to use for a test. This helps to easily identify which specimens should go in a particular tube. This is generally universal, although different manufacturers may utilize slightly different colors.

The colors of tube stoppers may be:

Lavender
Additive: Dipotassium EDTA (plastic tubes) or tripotassium EDTA (glass tubes).
Number of inversions: 8
Use: Whole-blood collection in hematologic tests; for donor screening.
Action: According to CLSI, dipotassium EDTA is superior to liquid tripotassium EDTA. Liquid EDTA dilutes the sample and results in falsely low blood count volumes.
Note: Do not use for coagulation tests; EDTA disrupts factor V and interferes with the thrombin-fibrinogen step. Must be filled up to the mark. This avoids excessive EDTA, which can shrink red cells, resulting in falsely low hematocrit, red cell indices and ESR.

Pink
Additive: Dipotassium EDTA (coated in plastic).
Number of inversions: 8
Use: Blood bank; crossmatching.

Note: A special label for blood bank; to avoid misidentification of patients.

Light Blue

Additive: Sodium citrate (3.2% or 3.8% Na citrate).
Blood volume: 4.5 mL
Number of inversions: 3 to 4; do not overmix (activates platelets).
Use: Coagulation tests.
Note: Sodium citrate can preserve labile clotting factors. Blood: Citrate ratio = 9:1; this ratio is critical; fill adequately.
Note: Requires centrifugation to use plasma for tests.
Special conditions: Polycythemia vera (hematocrit >55%) requires lower anticoagulant to prevent interference; use 3.2% Na citrate.

Light Blue (CTAD)

Additive: Sodium citrate, theophylline, adenosine and dipyridamole in glass.
Number of inversions: 3-4; do not overmix (it activates platelets).
Use: Platelet tests.
Note: VACUETTE® CTAD has a blue stopper and yellow top.

Green

Additive: Heparin with either Na, lithium or ammonium.
Number of inversions: 8
Use: Whole-blood chemistry determinations, STAT.
Action: Choose the correct additive; ammonium interferes with BUN tests and lithium interferes the least.
Note: Do not use for hematology tests; Wright's-stained heparinized blood shows a blue background.

Light Green with Green/Black Stoppers

Additive: Lithium heparin with gel (in a plasma separator tube).
Number of inversions: 8
Use: Tests for serum potassium.
Action: Heparin keeps potassium from leaking out of platelets during coagulation, while contamination from erythrocytes is avoided by the action of the separation gel.

Lime Green with Green/Black Stoppers

Additive: Lithium heparin with a mechanical separation device.
Number of inversions: 8
Use: Drug monitoring tests and zinc determinations.
Note: Tubes contain <50 microliters of zinc; avoids contamination.

Action: Mechanical separation device allows for only three minutes of centrifugation, which is faster than gel. Contamination by cells is reduced by over 50% than with gel.

Gray (Serum)
Additive: Na fluoride.
Number of inversions: 8
Use: Glucose determination, tests for lactic acid and alcohol levels.
Action: Sodium fluoride prevents glycolysis and stabilizes glucose for 24 hours.

Gray (Plasma)
Additive: Na fluoride with anticoagulant (potassium oxalate or disodium EDTA)
Number of inversions: 8
Use: Glucose determination, tests for lactic acid and alcohol levels.
Action: Sodium fluoride inhibits microbes' growth, which interferes with alcohol determination by producing alcohol as a by-product.
Note: Anticoagulant-containing tubes are used for plasma tests.

Royal Blue (Serum or Plain)
Additive: Silica.
Number of inversions: 8
Use: Toxin levels, analysis of trace metals and nutrient levels.
Note: Chemically clean with the least levels of metals; avoids contamination.

Royal Blue (Plasma)
Additive: Dipotassium EDTA or Na heparin.
Number of inversions: 8
Use: Toxin levels, analysis of trace metals and nutrient levels.
Note: Chemically clean with the least levels of metals; avoids contamination.

Tan
Additive: Dipotassium EDTA.
Number of inversions: 8
Use: Lead levels.
Note: Tubes contain <0.1 microgram per milliliter of lead; avoids contamination.

Yellow
Additive: ACD = acid citrate (anticoagulant) and dextrose.
Number of inversions: 8
Use: Blood bank cytology, HLA phenotype, DNA tests.

Action: Acid citrate provides anticoagulation by binding calcium, while dextrose stabilizes erythrocytes.

Yellow (SPS)

Additive: Sodium polyanethole sulfonate.
Number of inversions: 8
Use: Holds microbiology culture specimen.
Action: SPS provides anticoagulation by binding calcium and inhibits the destruction of microbes by preventing complement activation and phagocytosis.

Light Blue or Black (Glass) Cell Preparation Tube

Additive: Na citrate, gel, dense gradient fluid.
Number of inversions: 8
Use: Whole-blood molecular testing.
Action: Additives allow for mononuclear cells to be separated while transporting them in whole blood through the polyester gel and the density gradient fluid during centrifugation.

Red or Green Cell Preparation Tube

Additive: Na heparin, gel, dense gradient fluid.
Number of inversions: 8
Use: Whole-blood molecular testing; on tests requiring heparinized samples.

Black

Additive: Buffered citrate.
Number of inversions: 4
Use: Westergren sedimentation.
Note: Blood:citrate ratio = 4:1.

White or plasma preparation tubes

Additive: Dipotassium EDTA with a gel separator.
Number of inversions: 8
Use: Molecular diagnostic procedures.
Note: VACUETTE® has purple stoppers or white with yellow tops.

Orange

Additive: Thrombin.

Number of inversions: 8

Use: STAT chemistry tests; for use on patients taking anticoagulation meds.

Action: Thrombin is required for coagulation; adding it forms the clot in about five minutes.

Orange (Rapid Serum Tube)

Additive: Thrombin and a gel separator.

Number of inversions: 5

Use: STAT chemistry tests.

Action: Forms clot faster (five minutes); centrifuged to yield serum faster (10 minutes).

Red/Gray and Gold (Serum Separator Tubes)

Additive: Silica (to activate clot) and a gel separator.

Number of inversions: 5; to expose blood to the additive.

Use: Chemistry tests.

Action: Silica incites platelet activation; polymer barrier gel at the bottom changes viscosity while being centrifuged. This provides better separation of serum.

Note: Allow the clot to form completely (30 minutes) before centrifugation. Do not use for blood bank, immunoserology or drug testing.

Red

Additive: Silica (to activate clot).

Number of inversions: 5; to expose blood to the additive.

Use: Chemistry, blood bank and serology tests.

Action: Silica incites platelet activation; blood clots in 30 minutes.

Red (Glass) or Plain

Additive: None.

Number of inversions: 0

Use: Chemistry tests, blood bank and serology tests.

Action: Clots form through the normal coagulation pathways; blood clots in 60 minutes; centrifuge to yield serum.

Red/Light Gray; Clear; Discard

Additive: None.

Number of inversions: 0

Use: Collects discarded first draw (which may be falsely activated from trauma) for use in the winged collection or special factor assays.

Note: Tubes with a clot activator cannot replace these tubes; they are not required for routine coagulation (APTT or PT determinations).

Table of Blood Collection Tubes

COLOR	ADDITIVE	NUMBER OF INVERSIONS	DEPARTMENT OR TEST
Lavender	Ethylenediaminetetraacetic acid	8	H
Pink	Dipotassium EDTA	8	BB; crossmatching
White	Ethylenediaminetetraacetic acid with gel	8	MD
Light blue	Buffered Na citrate	3 to 4	CO
Gold or red/gray SST	Silica with gel to separate serum	5	C
Green	Heparin	8	C
Light green, green or black	Lithium heparin with gel	8	C
Green with a black or white ring	Lithium heparin with a mechanical separator	5 to 10	C
Red (silicone-coated, glass tube)	None	-	BB, C, I
Red with a black or white ring	Clot activator with or without gel	5 to 10	C, I
Orange	Thrombin & gel	8	C
Gray	K oxalate and Na fluoride	5 to 10	C
Gray	Na fluoride	5 to 10	C
Gray	Disodium EDTA and Na fluoride	8 to 10	
Tan	Dipotassium EDTA	8	Lead test
Royal blue	Na heparin	5 to 10	Toxicology
Yellow	Acid citrate dextrose	8	BB
Yellow	SPS	8	M
Black	Na citrate	4	H
Clear, Red, light gray	None	5 to 10	Discarding, storing or transportation

Legend: H – hematology; C – chemistry; BB – blood banking; CO – coagulation; I – immunoserology; M – microbiology; MD – molecular diagnostics

Order of Draw

The phlebotomist is often requisitioned to draw blood from one patient for use on different tests. To avoid erroneous results, blood must be collected in the proper sequence to prevent additives from carrying over to other tubes or contamination with tissue or microbes.

The Standard Order of Draw

1. Sterile tubes: Yellow (SPS) or blood culture tubes
2. Light blue
3. Serum tubes with or without gel: Red/gray, gold, red (plastic), red (glass) orange rapid serum tube, royal blue (clot activator)
4. Green, light green, royal blue (heparin)
4. Lavender, pink, royal blue (EDTA), tan
5. Gray
6. Yellow

By understanding the principles of additives, the phlebotomist knows that certain test results may be compromised by the wrong order of draw.

Light-blue-topped tubes are drawn before anticoagulant-containing tubes because carryover can falsely increase coagulation time. The physician might interpret these results and increase a patient's dosage of anticoagulant drugs.

EDTA (in lavender tubes) binds calcium and ferrous sulfate. EDTA contamination will falsely decrease calcium levels.

Contamination with Na citrate or potassium oxalate will falsely increase sodium and potassium levels.

Holding the tubes lower to fill them from the bottom avoids the carryover of additives.

Syringe

A syringe system may be needed for patients with smaller, more fragile veins. This is advantageous because the phlebotomist can manually control the pressure on the veins, unlike the automated filling on evacuated tubes, which is controlled by the vacuum.

Syringes are wrapped singly in sterile, disposable packaging.

Blood Transfer Device

When venipuncture is performed using the syringe system, blood needs to be transferred to the appropriate tubes immediately. Otherwise, a clot may form.

Do not puncture the stoppers with the syringe needle. Instead, a blood transfer device is more suitable. It consists of a holder with a needle. It looks like the ones used in the ETS.

To assemble the transfer device, insert the syringe into its hub. Each evacuated tube is then filled with the same order of draw as described above.

CLSI does not recommend this system for cobalt and chromium determinations since the plunger tip may contain these trace elements and contaminate the specimen.

The whole syringe and transfer device should be discarded into the sharps disposal.

Winged Blood Sets (Butterfly)

This is routinely used for IV infusions and venipuncture in the smaller and very fragile veins often encountered in cancer patients, small children and geriatric patients.

The butterfly needles are usually 21- to 23-gauge and are .50 to 0.75 inches long. An attachment resembling butterfly wings is used to hold the needle and secure the apparatus.

This is attached to a plastic tubing about 5 to 12 inches long with a hub that can attach to syringes or an ETS holder.

The winged blood collection system allows the phlebotomist to change the angle of venipuncture lower for more difficult veins.

However, these sets are more costly. They are generally reserved for problematic veins.

A discarded tube or an extra tube is needed to collect blood first. This removes air from the tube, which may otherwise underfill the first sample.

Sharps Disposal Containers

These are discussed earlier in the book.

Tourniquet

A tourniquet is a band of flat, disposable vinyl or nitrile applied around a limb. Its purpose is to occlude blood flow through the veins but not through an artery. This allows superficial veins to distend and become more palpable.

Vein Finders

Portable devices aid in locating veins, particularly in neonates, small children and geriatric patients.

The **Venoscope®** shines an intense LED light through the subcutaneous tissues, highlighting the veins, which absorb the light rays. The veins appear as dark lines. This enables the phlebotomist to delineate the veins for venipuncture. The **Neonatal Transilluminator** works the same way.

The **Wee-Sight Transilluminator** is used solely on an infant's skin since it produces no heat.

The **VEID**™ uses a beeping sensor activated by pressure changes. The beeping indicates that a needle has penetrated the vein and stops to indicate when a needle has exited the vein.

Gloves

It is mandatory to use gloves for a venipuncture procedure. They must be changed with every patient.

Use nonsterile gloves without powder routine procedures. Powder is avoided since it can contaminate the specimen and may cause latex allergy.

Handwashing or the use of alcohol-based hand rub is still required even when you are wearing gloves.

A cotton glove liner is available for phlebotomists with allergic dermatitis.

Additional Supplies

Skin cleansers, such as 70% isopropyl alcohol, are used to prevent microbial contamination during specimen collection.

For blood cultures, stronger solutions are required (see chapter 10).

Gauze is necessary for applying pressure to the wound after venipuncture. This prevents bleeding. Avoid cotton balls, since these can stick and often remove the platelet plug when taken off, rcinitiating the bleeding.

Bandages or **tape** are also used to apply pressure. **Self-adhesive gauze** is an alternative for those with allergies, excess bleeding or thin, frail skin (such as in geriatric patients). It is also used after an arterial blood collection, which requires more pressure to stop the bleeding.

Glass slides are used to create blood smears.

Biohazard bags, properly labeled and resistant to leaks, are used for specimen transport.

Alcohol-based hand rubs are used for hand hygiene. Cleansing the hands before putting gloves on and after taking gloves off is recommended.

Pens are necessary for labeling and noting down important information on the requisition forms.

Quality-Control Reminders

To ensure accurate test results, test equipment is regularly subjected to quality-control testing.

Disposable venipuncture equipment, such as syringes and needles, comes in well-sealed sterile packaging. Never use needles when the seal is broken.

Always inspect your materials for defects before performing a procedure. Check your needles for missing bevels or broken points.

Check your evacuated tubes for the expiration dates and discard expired tubes. Expired tubes may have already lost their vacuum, resulting in a short draw. This can interfere with test results.

On receiving a new lot of evacuated tubes:

- Draw water into one tube and measure the volume.
- Check additive-containing tubes for discoloration or contamination.
- Centrifuge a sample tube to test its stability.
- Cap and uncap one tube to check its stoppers.
- Document the quality-control results.
- Inform the manufacturer of any defects.
- Check if your syringe plungers are working.

Chapter 5: Routine Venipuncture

The CLSI has developed standards to ensure the quality of the venipuncture and, subsequently, the quality of the specimen and the reliability of the test results.

Step 1. Obtain a Requisition Form

Venipuncture begins when a phlebotomist receives the requisition form. This outlines the tests to be done on a patient as requested by a physician. This is part of the medical record and is considered a legal document. Every specimen collected must correspond with a requisition.

Requisition forms may be brought in by a patient from a doctor's clinic, received through the pneumatic tube or electronically encoded in the hospital information system.

The requisition form should always include the following:

- Patient identifiers: full name, age, gender and birth date; location
- Patient ID number (assigned by the hospital or the laboratory)
- Requesting physician's name and signature
- Test(s) requested
- Date and time of collection
- Urgency—whether STAT, routine or a timed collection
- Other information—billing codes or ICD Codes, special patient information (allergy to latex, fasting, areas to avoid for use in venipuncture)

The requisition form becomes your guide. This determines which tests to collect at which time and date on which patient. It is important to organize all the requisition forms at the start of your shift and before you do your sweeps. This ensures that you can collect all the needed samples with one venipuncture and determine patient preparation requirements, if any.

Step 2. Meet the Patient and Obtain Consent

When meeting patients, greet them with a smile. Give them your name and explain that you will collect specimens requested by their physician.

If questioned about which tests are requested and why, politely inform patients that this information is best given by their physicians.

Obtain permission to proceed with venipuncture. This may be verbal or nonverbal. Nonverbal consent is implied when patients roll up their sleeve or extend their arm.

In special situations, writing down the information or calling an interpreter to obtain consent may be necessary.

Step 3. Identify the Patient

This is the most important step. Serious errors and deaths can occur from misidentifying a patient.

CLSI standards require two identifiers. Ask every patient to verbally state their first and last names, spell them out and give their birth date. Compare these to the data on their ID bands with the requisition forms.

Pay attention to the ID numbers. Patients can have the same names, birth dates and physicians, but each has a unique ID number. High risks for misidentification include twins, neonates and names that sound similar.

In the outpatient setting, patients do not wear ID bands. Verify their information with proof of ID. ID cards with photographs are a requirement for legal tests.

For patients with impaired cognition, CLSI requires patient information to be provided by a caregiver, nurse or relative. You must document the informant's name on the requisition form as well.

Step 4. Prepare the Patient

Verify special preparations. These include appropriate fasting and skipping medications. In cases when the patient has not complied, report it to the nurse. If the nurse informs you that the physician still requires the specimen, document it on the requisition form and the specimen label as "not fasting."

Inquire about allergies to latex. If appropriate, switch to latex-free materials. Do not take latex supplies into the room of a patient with latex allergies.

Ask the patient to take a seat or sit up in bed. It is not recommended to draw blood while the patient is standing.

The proper position of the arm during venipuncture should be downward and extended, such that the wrists until the shoulder can be traced with a straight line. This way, your tubes may fill properly. Additive carryover is avoided as well. Do not hyperextend the elbows. This may make it difficult to find the veins.

You may ask the patient to support the elbow with a clenched fist of the opposite hand. This provides support for the procedure. In the outpatient laboratory, a phlebotomy wedge is placed in the same area to support the arm.

Reassure the patient throughout the procedure. Never promise that it will be painless. Stay alert to the patient's condition. Some patients may faint. If they say they feel faint, have them lie down for the venipuncture. A small pillow or a rolled-up towel may help support and position the arm.

Importantly, avoid falls. Make sure the seats have barriers that may catch a fainting patient. If you have lowered a bed rail, always return it before leaving the patient.

Before venipuncture, ask patients to remove any objects, gum or a thermometer from their mouths. When they have been eating or drinking, wait until they have swallowed before you proceed. Patients can accidentally choke on food or other items during the venipuncture.

Step 5. Select Your Equipment

Place your supply tray within reach of your free hand. It should lie on a stable surface.

Never put this on the patient's bed; it may fall and spill. Do not place it in a patient's eating space either, as it is unsanitary.

At this point, recheck the requisition form. Take your blood collection system (ETS, syringes or butterflies) and the necessary tubes.

A butterfly system is preferable for patients who are very young or very old with fragile veins. For patients with small and thin veins, the syringe system may be a better choice. Also, consider the number of tests needed and the volume of blood to be extracted.

Visualize each supply and read the expiration dates. Discard opened needle packages and expired tubes.

Set the tubes in your working area in proper order. Additional tubes should also be within reach.

Step 6. Perform Hand Hygiene and Wear Gloves

Perform hand hygiene with alcohol-based hand gel in front of the patient. Apply a pair of gloves.

Changing gloves between patients is an OSHA mandate.

Pull these over the cuffs of your lab coat or protective gown. This minimizes any areas of contact with your bare skin.

Step 7. Apply Tourniquets Properly

A tourniquet allows the veins to distend by obstructing venous return. It is not strong enough to impede arteries. This helps with locating the venipuncture site and makes blood collection easier, as blood has been allowed to pool.

However, leaving the tourniquet on too long causes hemolysis. This results in inaccurate test results. The tourniquet should be used for only a maximum of one minute.

Following this principle, you will often apply the tourniquet twice—when choosing the venipuncture site and also right before you draw blood. CLSI recommends waiting for at least two minutes before reapplying the tourniquet.

Ideally, a new disposable, latex-free tourniquet is used for each patient. This avoids BBP and microbial transmission.

To Apply a Tourniquet Properly

1. Choose a site on the arm at least three or four inches superior to the antecubital fossa or the site for venipuncture. The tourniquet should be applied to a muscle rather than a joint or bony area. It may be applied over gauze or clothes to avoid discomfort.

2. Place the tourniquet flat around the patient's arm, ensuring it is centered. Grasp both ends and pull to create tension. Tuck one side under the other to form a downward-facing loop. The free end should be away from the antecubital fossa.

3. Make sure the tourniquet is not too tight. This may obstruct blood flow. Small pinpoint red lesions (petechiae) and skin blanching near the tourniquet are signs that the tourniquet is too tight. You should still be able to feel the radial pulse.

Do not ask your patient to pump the fist. This causes hemoconcentration. This action is ideal for blood donation but not for laboratory testing. Hemoconcentration can affect test results.

After applying the tourniquet, veins are found on sight or palpated by your index finger. Veins feel rubbery or spongy and cylindrical. You can feel the vein's direction or orientation and depth. Unlike arteries, veins should not have a pulse.

Select the vein that is large and palpable.

You may find a visual landmark, such as a mole or skin crease, or you may mark the site with the corner of an alcohol pad.

You must keep your gloves on during this process to avoid transmitting microbes.

Remember to avoid hemolysis. Remove the tourniquet swiftly after choosing your site. The selection process should take only a minute.

To Remove a Tourniquet Properly
Pull the free end to release.

Step 8. Choose the Site

Venipuncture sites are preferably at the antecubital fossa, which is anterior and inferior to the elbow crease. As described in chapter 3, this area is where you can find three superficial veins most appropriate for the procedure. In descending order of preference, these are the median cubital, cephalic and basilic veins.

The **median cubital vein** is preferred since it is larger and well-anchored. It lies in the center of the antecubital area. It is the least painful site since this vein overlies aponeurosis.

CLSI states that both arms must be inspected to locate this vein before choosing another vein.

The **cephalic vein** is the second choice. It is the most lateral, and it can be difficult to locate. It is also less well-anchored. When choosing this as the venipuncture site, avoid puncturing laterally since it is close to the lateral cutaneous nerve.

The **basilic vein** is the least well-anchored of the three veins. It is on the medial aspect of the antecubital area. It is moveable and tends to roll away when a needle is inserted.

This contributes to hematoma. This is the last choice and is often discouraged because it is nearer the nerves and brachial artery. This site causes more complications and complaints than any other vein.

When no other vein is available and you must puncture the basilic vein, take care to palpate for the brachial pulse. Avoid accidentally puncturing the brachial artery.

Some techniques to make the veins more prominent may be employed.

- Massage the patient's forearm, moving up from the wrist to the elbow.
- Ask the patient to hang their arm down the side of the chair briefly.
- Apply a warm compress to the area for about five minutes.

These superficial veins may be traced up to the wrists, although this is unsuitable for venipuncture since the veins are smaller and more mobile. Punctures near the wrists cause more pain. Punctures near the palmar and lateral areas of the wrists carry a high risk of puncturing an artery, nerves or tendons. CLSI recommends against this.

Small superficial veins are also found on the dorsum of the hand. These may be suitable for venipuncture. Smaller needles or butterfly sets are used to collect blood from this area. Often, this area is reserved for IV lines.

Step 9. Cleanse the Site

Routinely, 70% isopropyl alcohol on a presoaked pad is used to prepare the site for the venipuncture. Rub two to three inches around the venipuncture site in a to-and-fro motion. If the patient's arm is still visibly soiled, repeat with a new alcohol pad.

Wait about one minute for the alcohol to dry. Do not touch the site or fan or wipe it. Drying maximizes the bacteriostatic action of alcohol.

Puncturing a site while the alcohol is still wet causes a stinging sensation, and contamination might cause hemolysis of the specimen.

If you palpate the vein again, you must repeat the skin cleansing afterward.

Step 10. Assemble Your Devices In Front of the Patient

As the alcohol is drying, recheck your equipment. Make sure everything is within reach. Assemble your blood collection devices (whether ETS, butterfly or syringe systems) in front of the patient.

Step 11. Puncture the Site

Apply the tourniquet once again. You may ask the patient to make a fist but without pumping it.

Hold your ETS holder firmly. Your thumb should be above the holder while your other fingers are under it. At this point, uncap the needle and examine the point for a missing bevel or a bent end. Discard defective needles.

Position the needle with the bevel up. With the thumb of your nondominant hand, pull the skin about one to two inches below and slightly lateral to the site. This keeps it taut around the selected vein. It helps to keep the vein firmly in place and prevents it from rolling.

Do not anchor the vein with your thumb and index finger above the site. Any sudden movement, especially in a noncooperative patient, can cause accidental needle pricks on these fingers.

Hold the ETS properly close to the hub. Position the needle in line with the vein. The needle bevel should be facing upward at a 15°-to-30° angle. Insert the needle through the skin smoothly and swiftly with one motion. When it has entered the vein, you can feel the resistance lowering.

Secure the ETS holder with your fingers braced on the patient's arm while you insert the evacuated tubes to collect blood.

Instruct the patient to open the fist as blood flows down the tube. If blood collection could last more than a minute, release the tourniquet with your free hand.

Blood is collected with the tubes at a downward angle. This avoids additive carryover from the needle. Follow the proper order of drawing.

Make sure each tube fills to its fill mark. If it does not fill, the tube may have already lost its vacuum. This may happen even though it has not yet expired. Discard this tube and use a new one. This illustrates the importance of having spare tubes within reach.

Invert each tube the appropriate number of times immediately after filling it. These few seconds do not cause any significant discomfort to your patient. They also ensure the integrity of the specimen.

When you are on your final tube, take it out and invert it appropriately. Only then should you remove the needle from the patient. This prevents blood spills from the needle and prevents BBP transmission.

Make sure the tourniquet is released before removing the needle.

Some needle devices activate before the needle is removed from the patient. Otherwise, place a piece of clean gauze over the needle, remove the needle swiftly and smoothly, then activate the safety device.

Step 12. Apply Pressure over the Puncture Site

Make sure the needle is out of the vein before applying any pressure.

Keep pressure on the site with a clean gauze, or, if the patient is capable, ask them to hold down the gauze for about two to three minutes.

Bending the elbow is not advisable. It does not provide enough pressure to prevent blood from leaking into the tissues. This causes hematoma.

Step 13. Discard Sharps

Do not attempt to disassemble the blood collection systems. Discard the entire used ETS needle and holder into the sharps container.

Step 14. Label Each Tube While the Patient Is Still in the Room

Label each tube with your indelible pen or stick electronically generated labels. Note the time of collection on the tubes.

You must make sure the following information is on the labels:

- Patient identifiers: given name and last name
- ID number (admitted patients) or birth date (for outpatients)
- Your initials
- Date and time collected

Specimens for the blood bank need additional information. This is found on the patient's blood bank ID band.

You must label each tube right after collecting the specimen and before leaving the patient. Carefully compare your labels with the patient's ID band.

You may show your labels to the patient and verbally ask for confirmation as an additional identifying step.

Mislabeling the specimen is just as harmful as improperly identifying a patient.

To transport specimens through the pneumatic tubes, pack the tubes and their corresponding requisition forms in a biohazard bag.

Some tubes require special handling (see chapter 11); place these in appropriate containers immediately after labeling.

Step 15. Watch Out for Adverse Reactions

At this point, continue to monitor the patient for immediate adverse reactions.

During these five minutes, the venipuncture site should no longer bleed. Examine the site for about 5 to 10 seconds (to comply with CLSI standards), then apply an adhesive bandage.

These steps are necessary to prevent hematoma. A hematoma from subcutaneous bleeding can result in a severe nerve compression injury. The phlebotomist may be held liable for these injuries.

To prevent reactions to latex or adhesive in allergic patients, paper tape is available.

Self-adhesive gauze is an alternative for those with allergies, excess bleeding or thin, frail skin (such as in geriatric patients).

In some patients with a higher risk for bleeding, added pressure may be applied with a folded gauze bandage or secured with a gauzelike material.

Instruct patients that bandages may be removed after 15 minutes. They should avoid lifting items for at least an hour.

Step 16. Discard Used Supplies

Collect all used supplies and discard these in the appropriate containers. Remove your gloves and discard these as well. Perform hand hygiene.

Step 17. Thank the Patient

Return the bed rail if you had lowered it. This makes sure the patient does not fall. Forgetting to do so may subject you to legal issues.

Thank the patient as you leave the room.

Once you have completed the above steps in the outpatient laboratory, patients can be released. Be sure to thank them for cooperating. Remind them to eat and drink if they have been fasting and have no other procedures for the day.

Clean up your work area before the next patient.

Step 18. Deliver the Specimen

Only when you have successfully sent the specimen to the laboratory can you consider your work completed. You may also need to complete the paperwork. This may vary depending on your workplace protocols.

Timely delivery and proper handling of specimens are as important as performing the venipuncture successfully. Some guidelines include:

- Deliver specimens as soon as possible.
- STAT tests take priority.
- Secure your properly packed specimen for the pneumatic tubes. Verify that the specimen has gone through the tube before leaving the area.
- Tubes with gel separators must remain upright to activate clotting and avoid hemolysis.
- Tubes with anticoagulant additives must be centrifuged within two hours.
- The ideal time for the specimen to reach the laboratory department should be within 45 minutes. This allows time for immediate centrifugation.

Some tests are especially sensitive to improper transport and processing.

- Glucose determinations are affected by glycolysis, which causes falsely low values.
- Potassium assays are sensitive to hemolysis, which leaks potassium out of the cells and causes falsely high serum values.
- Coagulation factors may be labile to temperature. Leaving the specimen at room temperature for a long time causes these to be destroyed, causing erroneous results.

Chapter 6: Venipuncture Complications and Special Situations

Possible complications may arise with each step of venipuncture. As the phlebotomist, you must always be wary of situations when you may need to adjust the procedure.

Outlined below are each step of venipuncture with emphasis on difficult situations and avoidable complications.

Step 1. Obtain a Requisition Form

The emergency department often telephones the laboratory to request a phlebotomist. Labels are printed automatically.

At the emergency department, you must obtain a completed requisition form before you locate the patient and perform the venipuncture.

Step 2. Meet the Patient and Obtain Consent

Sleeping Patients

You must wake sleeping patients politely. Identify yourself and wait for them to be oriented. Ask them to identify themselves verbally and to consent to the procedure. Remember, you can face legal issues for venipuncture without consent.

Comatose Patients

Greet comatose patients as though they were conscious. Often, patients in a coma are still able to hear, understand and remember despite being unable to respond.

In this situation, a nurse in charge or a family member will be present to identify the patient and give consent.

Psychiatric Wards

In this area, it is better to ask a nurse to assist you. The patients are usually anxious and will be reassured by the presence of a familiar person, such as the nurse.

Remember to keep your equipment far from these patients' reach.

Other People in the Room

When **health care providers** or **clergy** are with a patient, it is better to return after they have left. However, if you are there for a timed collection or a STAT test, explain the urgency and ask for permission to proceed with the venipuncture.

Greet **visitors** and **relatives** warmly. Allow them to leave the room for the procedure. If they choose to stay, you may pull the curtains around the bed. Visitors or **parents** are helpful when dealing with pediatric or very anxious patients.

Patients Not in Their Rooms

Locate them through the nurse. They may just be walking around or could have been taken to radiology or other units. If you need to draw blood for a timed specimen or a STAT test, it may be necessary to go to the unit where the patient was taken.

Otherwise, inform the nurse to reschedule the test or alert the laboratory when the patient is available. Note this appropriately on the requisition form.

Step 3. Identify the Patient

Missing Wrist or Ankle Bands

In this case, find the nurse to replace the bands before you draw blood. In some facilities, a nurse may be allowed to sign the requisition slip to verify the patient's identity.

Psychiatric Wards

In psychiatric wards, ID bands are often not worn per facility protocols. In this case, you must identify patients per outpatient laboratory protocols. Ask them to verbally state their first and last names, spell them out and give their birth date.

For patients with cognitive impairment, CLSI requires patient information to be provided by a caregiver, nurse or relative. You must document their name on the requisition form.

Unknown Patients or John Does

In the emergency department, patients may arrive unidentified. The American Association of Blood Banks requires each unidentified patient to receive a **temporary ID**. Some facilities use a temporary name (such as John Doe) with a number.

After the patient is identified, the facility can issue a unique patient ID number. Take note of the temporary ID on the requisition slip and cross-reference it with the permanent ID number once it becomes available.

Cognitive Impairments and Language Barriers

For patients who are too young, have cognitive impairments or cannot speak English, CLSI requires patient information to be provided by a caregiver. In some instances, the nurse may verify the patient's identity. You must document the informant's name on the requisition form.

Step 4. Patient Preparation

Pre-examination variables are those that may affect the integrity of the specimens and alter test results. Nurses or providers must carefully instruct the patients of restrictions before blood collection. The phlebotomist must verify that the patient has complied before proceeding with the venipuncture.

Basal State

It is preferable to obtain specimens during the basal state. This is when the patient is well-rested and has fasted (no food or drinks except water for the last 12 hours). This is often early in the morning.

This is because test reference ranges were established from a set of randomly selected normal subjects in the basal state. While not every test is affected by strenuous activity and fasting, venipuncture during the basal state achieves the best comparison of patient test values with reference ranges.

This also means that the early morning is the busiest hour for the phlebotomist. Many tests can still be obtained throughout the day.

Diet

Eating and drinking affect tests for blood sugar and triglycerides.

Blood glucose spikes immediately after eating and returns to baseline in about two hours.

When blood is collected too soon after a meal (especially one of fried, greasy food and dairy), it may appear cloudy. This is termed ***lipemia,*** referring to the high lipid content of the blood sample. This interferes with test results.

Alcohol intake increases blood sugar transiently.

Chronic alcohol intake affects hepatic assays for ALT and AST. It raises triglyceride, estrogen and luteinizing hormone, prolactin, catecholamines, cholesterol, HDL, aldosterone and iron levels. It reduces testosterone levels as well.

Caffeine increases levels of gastrin, ACTH, cortisol, fatty acids, lipoprotein and glycerol.

Fasting

The following analytes are affected by a **nonfasted state**: blood glucose, lipid panel, growth hormone, AST, bilirubin, phosphorus, uric acid and blood urea nitrogen.

A **prolonged fasted state** causes bilirubin, glucagon, triglycerides, fatty acids, lactate and assays for ketones to be elevated. This state also lowers values for cholesterol, free thyroid hormones, glucose and insulin levels.

Since diet can affect so many tests, certain assays require fasting. You must verify if the patient has complied with the necessary eight to 12 hours of fasting. If not, report it to the nurse. If the nurse confirms that the physician still requires the specimen, document it on both the requisition form and the specimen label as "not fasting."

Postural Changes

Changes in a position may affect tests that measure protein-bound compounds.

Moving abruptly from a supine to an upright posture shifts water from the plasma into the tissues. Since protein is too large to pass through blood vessel walls, the sample obtained may be falsely concentrated.

The results of the following tests are significantly increased by 5% to 15% within only 10 minutes of changing positions: bilirubin, calcium, lipid panel, renin and aldosterone and enzymatic determinations.

It takes about 30 minutes for these analytes to return to their baseline values after the patient lies back down.

For lipid panel tests, patients are instructed to remain recumbent or sit down for at least five minutes before venipuncture.

Importantly, values for renin and aldosterone and catecholamines can increase to twice their original values in an hour after shifting positions. For such tests, patients are instructed to stay recumbent for at least 30 minutes before blood is drawn. This is especially required for patients with congestive heart failure and hepatic disorder.

Additionally, you must note down the patient's position during venipuncture on the requisition forms.

Exercise

Exercise affects laboratory values. This depends on the extent of vigorous activity, the patient's body type and muscle mass and the timing of blood collection.

Following **short-term exercise**, results are increased for creatinine, creatine kinases, fatty acid, aldosterone, angiotensin, bilirubin, HDL, AST, lactic acid, insulin, lactate dehydrogenase, uric acid, hormone assays, renin, potassium and white blood cell counts. Results are lowered for arterial blood pH and PCO_2.

Immediately after strenuous exercise, clotting factors, platelets and cholesterol levels are transiently increased.

Moderate exercise elevates creatinine, potassium, lactate, metabolic byproducts, hormones, bilirubin, insulin and uric acid levels. It decreases arterial pH and partial pressure of carbon dioxide.

Acute and regular exercise (such as by bodybuilders) have varying effects on laboratory assays.

Acute exercise may activate anaerobic glycolysis, resulting in elevated metabolic byproducts, such as aspartate aminotransferases, lactate dehydrogenase and creatine kinases. The white cell count increases as they are released from the vessel walls during exercise.

These values typically return to baseline after a few hours except for muscle enzyme levels and renin and aldosterone. These may remain increased for up to 24 hours.

Prolonged exercise results in a more prolonged elevation of metabolic byproducts, such as aspartate aminotransferases, lactate dehydrogenase and creatine kinases, as well as hormones.

Stress

Stress, possibly induced by anxiety and fear of needles, transiently increases catecholamine, cortisol, adrenocorticotropic hormone levels and white cell counts.

In **crying children**, white cell count elevates as a response to sympathetic stimulation. This returns to normal only after an hour of calming down.

In contrast, white cell levels determined during the basal state are lower until the patient resumes normal daily activities.

Panic attacks may result in hyperventilation and interfere with arterial blood gas results. Consequently, lactate and fatty acids are elevated.

Smoking

Nicotine interferes with laboratory assays depending on the kind and number of cigarettes. Acutely, nicotine elevates catecholamines, cortisol, growth hormones and lipid levels. Blood glucose and urea nitrogen may elevate by up to 10%.

Prolonged effects of nicotine include hemoconcentration (increased hemoglobin, red cell count and MCV) and affect immunity by lowering immunoglobulin levels.

Altitude

At higher altitudes, oxygen levels are lower. This causes higher counts of hemoglobin and hematocrit. Thus, a different set of normal values is used for individuals living at higher altitudes.

Age and Sex

Age affects laboratory tests due to changes in fluid composition.

Levels of hormones and body mass composition differ between male and female patients. Males usually have higher levels of hemoglobin and hematocrit.

Reference ranges are varied for each subset of patients.

Pregnancy

Pregnancy causes multiple biological changes in a woman's body. Notably, plasma volume rises and dilutes the values for laboratory tests. Red cell count, total protein, ALP, estrogen, fatty acids and serum iron levels are decreased. Pregnancy is a pro-inflammatory state, which may also increase erythrocyte sedimentation rates and certain clotting factors.

Fever

Fever elevates insulin and glucagon.

Malnutrition

- Results are increased for these tests:
    - Ketones, lactic acids, bilirubin, triglycerides
- Results are decreased for these tests:
    - Glucose, serum albumin, protein, free thyroid hormones

Diurnal Variation

This is the normal fluctuation of hormones and metabolites throughout the day. It is affected by sleep, activity, arousal levels, light and darkness.

Thyroid-stimulating hormones and cortisol levels are notably sensitive to diurnal variations. There can be about a 50% difference in levels between an 8 a.m. sample and a 4 p.m. sample.

Diurnal variations affect tests in the following way:

- Results are increased for these tests:
    - Cortisol, bilirubin, aldosterone

    - Hemoglobin, serum iron, potassium
    - Thyroid-stimulating hormone, hormone assays
- Results are decreased for these tests:
    - Creatinine, phosphate, blood glucose, triglycerides
    - Eosinophil counts

Medications

Certain drugs interfere with laboratory results by either interfering with the assay procedure or altering the patient's metabolism.

Common medications and their possible effects are listed below:

MEDICATIONS	TESTS INCREASED	TESTS DECREASED
Antibiotics	ALT, AST, bilirubin, blood urea nitrogen, creatinine	*None*
Aspirin, herbal medicines	Prothrombin time, bleeding time	*None*
Chemotherapeutic agents	*None*	All blood cell lines (RBC, WBC and platelet)
Corticosteroids, estrogen	Amylase, lipase	*None*
Dyslipidemic drugs	Prothrombin time, APTT	*None*
Diuretics	Calcium, blood sugar, uric acid	Sodium, potassium
Fluorescein dyes	Creatinine, cortisol	*None*
Opioids	ALT, AST, pancreatic enzymes	*None*
Oral contraceptive pills	*None*	Cholesterol, triglycerides, HDL, luteinizing hormone, follicle-stimulating hormone, serum iron, ESR
Paracetamol	ALT, AST, bilirubin	

These medications may need to be discontinued for at least four hours and up to 24 hours for blood tests.

Other Procedures

When a patient is subjected to a procedure, make note of it on your requisition slips (such as ongoing blood transfusion), as this can affect test results as well.

Adverse Reactions

Needle phobia occurs in 10% of people. This is an irrational and intense fear at the sight of a needle. It can be so severe as to lead to fatal cardiac arrhythmia. These patients are highly sensitive to the needle prick. They may faint, be diaphoretic or complain of nausea or dizziness. For these patients, make sure that an emergency cart is nearby.

Fainting or **syncope** is due to a sudden decrease in blood flow to the brain. The heart rate and blood pressure drop. This is followed by a sudden loss of consciousness. This is also known as the **vasovagal response.** This may be triggered by the sight of needles and blood, fear, pain, prolonged exertion or intense heat. Other causes are orthostatic hypotension, hypoglycemia, heart conditions, anemia or CNS disorders.

Patients often appear pale, hyperventilating, cold and clammy just before fainting. They may complain of dizziness, blurring or tunneling of vision and nausea. Be wary of these symptoms. Always make sure that barriers, such as armrests and bed rails, are around to prevent fall injuries.

Early-morning patients who have not yet eaten or drunk are prone to syncope. When your patient shows symptoms of fainting before the procedure, instruct them to breathe deeply, clench and unclench their thighs, turn their ankles gently clockwise and counterclockwise or do other distracting actions.

If your patient has fainted, immediately release the tourniquet. Withdraw the needle and apply pressure to the venipuncture site. While doing this, call for help.

In the outpatient setting, recline the patient and lower their head. Be careful that they do not fall.

If they regain consciousness, instruct them to breathe deeply and do distracting actions. Have the patient lie down and loosen tight clothing. A cold compress may be applied to the forehead and nape. This helps revive them. Spirit of ammonia is no longer recommended.

Notify the first-aid staff. All syncope incidents must be documented per facility protocol.

For those outpatients who have fasted and feel faint, let them have a sweet drink if you have succeeded in collecting blood and they have no other procedures. Ask them to stay in the facility for about 15 to 30 minutes of observation. Notify the first-aid staff.

While it is rare, **seizures** may be triggered by venipuncture. When a patient suddenly starts having jerky movements and is unresponsive, immediately release the tourniquet and withdraw the needle. Apply pressure to the venipuncture site. While doing this, call for help.

Make sure the patient is safe from possible injuries. Turn their head to one side. Do not attempt to place any object in their mouth. Do not leave the patient.

Inform the physician if the patient's seizing caused deep punctures on the venipuncture site.

The time of seizure onset and duration must be documented per facility protocol.

If you are in the outpatient laboratory, make sure the patient has been examined by a physician or first-aid staff before they leave the facility.

Nausea and/or **vomiting** may occur at any time during or after venipuncture. When the patient informs you of being nauseated, have a basin and washcloth ready. You may also instruct the patient to take slow, deep breaths and apply a cold compress to the forehead. Notify the first-aid staff.

Observe patients for changes in conditions as well. Notify the nurses when you notice infiltrated IV lines, shortness of breath, changes in sensorium and, in some cases, an expired patient. See chapter 15 for cardiopulmonary resuscitation procedures.

When faced with a situation where a **patient refuses to have blood extracted** even after you have explained it, you cannot force it. You could be charged with battery. Therefore, you must inform the nurses, who can still try to convince the patient. When all these efforts fail, document the patient's refusal on the requisition form.

Step 5. Select Your Equipment

Inquire for any allergies, especially to latex. If appropriate, switch to latex-free materials. Be careful not to take latex supplies into the room of a patient with latex allergies.

A patient may be allergic to adhesives on the bandage or skin cleansers. Have paper tape and alternative skin cleansers ready.

Step 6. Perform Hand Hygiene and Wear Gloves

Step 7. Apply Tourniquets Properly

It is recommended that a tourniquet be used for a maximum of one minute. Leaving a tourniquet on longer causes **hemoconcentration**, which increases protein-bound substances in the blood. It affects tests determining lipids, proteins and red blood cells. It also affects analytes transported through proteins, such as iron and other minerals.

Hemoconcentration is also caused by excessively probing the needle on the site, venipuncture on sclerotic veins or edematous limbs and pumping fists.

Remind your patients not to pump their fists, especially when drawing blood for lactic acid assays and potassium determinations. This causes potassium to increase by 20% and blood pH to lower.

A prolonged tourniquet also causes **hemolysis**, which leaks potassium, lactate and certain enzymes out of the cell.

Leaving the tourniquet for two minutes elevates cholesterol by up to 5% and as high as 15% after only five minutes.

After one minute, hemoglobin increases by 3%; after three minutes, it increases by 7%.

Always follow the CLSI's standards of using a tourniquet for only a maximum of one minute.

Step 8. Choose the Site

When no other arm or hand veins are suitable, the lower limb veins can be used. Obtain permission from the physician first. These veins are more prone to infections and thrombi.

Do not perform venipuncture in areas with possible infections, contamination or low blood flow, such as over hematomas and on edematous limbs and sclerosed veins. These may potentially alter test results or cause significant discomfort to patients.

Avoid the Following Areas:

Certain veins may have a **thrombus** or be already **sclerosed** (or hardened) from the stress of multiple punctures (i.e., in patients receiving chemotherapeutic drugs or IV drug abusers). They are occluded and may have poor circulation, which can alter test results.

A **hematoma** forms when blood leaks out from the veins and accumulates in the tissues. It appears like a bruise. Venipuncture in this area is uncomfortable and causes you to draw out hemolyzed blood from tissues.

When no other veins are suitable except for one near a hematoma, always puncture inferior to the hematoma. This ensures a sample of circulating blood.

Specimens from **edematous limbs** alter laboratory results. It may be contaminated with tissue fluid. Edema is a consequence of fluid retention caused by cardiac, renal or hepatic diseases, inflammation or infections. It is also commonly due to infiltration from the IV fluid. Alert the nurse in charge when you notice an infiltrated IV line.

Often, patients have **IV fluids** in their arm veins. First, locate a suitable vein on the opposite arm to avoid contamination. Otherwise, you may draw blood inferior to the IV infusion point and, if possible, from another vein. Dermal punctures are preferred.

CLSI standards state to ask the nurse to interrupt the IV infusion for about two minutes before the venipuncture. Document the situation on the requisition form as "specimen collected below the IV infusion point."

Avoid venipuncture on areas with **nonintact skin**, such as those **with a burn, scar** or **tattoo**. New or swollen tattoos are prone to infections. Areas with a healed burn or scar have poorer blood circulation, which may alter results.

Do not apply a tourniquet or attempt venipuncture on the arm on the side of a recent **mastectomy**. Lymph nodes may have been dissected during mastectomy, obstructing the lymphatic circulation. This causes higher levels of lymphocytes and byproducts. It also makes patients prone to **lymphedema**. The risks increase when a tourniquet is applied to this area. This site is more prone to infection when punctured due to the absence of lymph nodes.

In patients recovering from a **bilateral mastectomy**, consult their physician before you attempt a venipuncture. The patient's hand or fingers may still be suitable sites.

On **obese** patients, you may need to use a blood pressure cuff or longer bariatric-type tourniquets to locate their veins. Avoid probing. It is not only painful, but it can hemolyze the sample. A syringe system with a longer needle may be an alternative.

Patients undergoing **hemodialysis** often have an arteriovenous graft or fistula on either arm. It is made by surgically fusing a radial artery with a cephalic vein. This is a venous access device. It is more prone to infection and prolonged bleeding. The patients may also have a temporary catheter accessing a large vein, usually the internal jugular or femoral veins. Only trained staff can draw blood from these areas.

You must first be sure that the arm has no grafts or fistulas before you apply a tourniquet. Compressing the vessels of these arms can compromise the integrity of these devices. Draw blood only on the arm without an arteriovenous graft or fistula.

Step 9. Cleanse the Site

Remember, do not use isopropyl alcohol to cleanse the skin for venipuncture to collect blood for alcohol levels. This can potentially interfere with the results (See chapter 11).

Step 10. Assemble Your Devices in Front of the Patient

An exemption to this rule is for pediatric patients. Devices are assembled out of their view to minimize anxiety.

Step 11. Puncture the Site

When unable to draw blood, you may be able to remedy the situation without having to do another puncture. Be sure to check for the following:

Needle Position

Having the needle **bevel too close to the vessel wall** obstructs blood flow. Make sure to insert at the recommended 15°-to-30°-angle. An angle that is too narrow positions the bevel too close to the upper vessel wall. An angle that is too steep positions the bevel too close to the lower vessel wall.

Failure to insert the bevel facing upward obstructs blood flow. To remedy this, remove the evacuated tube and pull the needle slowly. When it is just underneath the skin, rotate the needle about one-quarter of a turn. This fixes the bevel position and allows you to adjust your angle so that blood may flow into the tubes.

The needle is advanced too deep into the vein. When using the ETS, you must firmly brace the holder as you insert or change the tubes. If you fail to do so, the needle may puncture through the vein into the tissues. This obstructs blood flow and can cause hematoma.

Slowly pulling the needle may remedy this situation. Be sure to apply additional pressure later to reduce the risk of hematoma.

The needle angle is too narrow. When inserting too close to the skin, you may initially reach the lumen of the vein successfully, but blood will flow too slowly into the collecting tube. This angle allows blood to leak into the tissues. This may create hematoma.

You can remedy this by gently advancing the needle until blood flows more freely. However, if a hematoma forms, immediately discontinue the venipuncture and then apply pressure.

The needle is not inside the vein. When you cannot anchor the site firmly, the vein may have rolled and the needle now lies next to the vein. Palpate the vein and needle gently.

You may remedy this by slowly withdrawing the needle until you see its bevel just underneath the skin. Anchor the vein and redirect your needle. You must first establish the vein location; never probe blindly. Do not probe vigorously. This causes pain and enlarges the puncture site. It may cause hematoma or an accidental arterial injury.

Collapsed Vein

The vein collapses when too much pressure is applied to it, such as when:

- The ETS is too large.
- A syringe plunger was pulled too hard and fast.
- A tourniquet was applied too tightly.
- A tourniquet was applied too near the venipuncture site.

When this happens, release the tourniquet, remove the evacuated tube or release the plunger. Retry with a tube requiring lesser volume. If these techniques do not work, you will need to perform another puncture with a smaller needle through the syringe system or a butterfly set.

Faulty Evacuated Tubes

Some tubes may have lost their vacuum due to expiration, manufacturing errors or accidental punctures. They do not collect blood properly. When you suspect this, you should use a new tube.

Partially Filled Tubes

An improperly filled tube is unacceptable for certain tests, especially when the tests are sensitive to blood:additive ratios.

- Excess anticoagulant in light-blue tubes dilutes the plasma and increases coagulation time.
- Excess EDTA in a lavender tube shrinks erythrocytes, resulting in falsely low hematocrit, red cell indices and ESR.
- Incompletely filled gray tubes cause hemolysis.

An SST and red tubes are not affected by the fill level. These tubes must be filled with enough volume to run the necessary tests.

A partial-draw tube is an alternative for instances when a full tube cannot be obtained. They require less volume and have a mark indicating the proper fill level.

Selecting Another Site

When you cannot remedy the problems listed above, you should attempt another venipuncture either in another arm or below the first site. Always use a new needle.

When the second attempt is unsuccessful, do not try a third. Notify the nurse and request another phlebotomist to collect the specimen.

Complications from the Venipuncture Procedure

Nerve damage is the most severe complication of venipuncture. The most critical nerve to avoid is the **median antebrachial cutaneous nerve.** Injuries to this nerve are often permanent. Complications include weakness, loss of sensation and motor function and chronic pain.

You can be alerted to this if the patient complains of tingling, shock-like sensations or overt pain and numbness. Immediately discontinue venipuncture.

This complication is preventable by following the proper venipuncture techniques. Always avoid probing blindly or vigorously, inserting in a lateral direction and sudden movements.

But when it occurs, apply a cold compress to the site. Instruct the patient or request the nurse to use a warm compress after a few hours. Report the incident to the nurse for medical attention and properly document it per your facility's protocols.

Iatrogenic anemia can be induced by removing too much blood in a short period. Infants and geriatric patients are more prone to this, as they often have smaller blood volumes. Extract only the minimum volume from these patients.

In newborns, blood collection is monitored in the first 24 hours of life. The blood extracted should not exceed 3% of their blood volume at any given time and should not exceed 10% of their blood volume in one month. The patient's chart also contains a log of blood collection volumes.

A child's blood volume is estimated using the following formula:

Blood volume in milliliters = weight in kilograms x 100

Therefore, a newborn weighing 3 kg has a blood volume of 300 mL. Blood collection should not exceed 9 mL at any given time and 30 mL in one month.

Select the equipment for pediatric patients to collect the least blood volume possible. A 23-gauge butterfly needle connected to a syringe system may be used on small children. Whenever possible, a dermal puncture with microcollection tubes is preferable.

An ETS using pediatric tubes, which collect a minimum of 1.8 mL, is acceptable for older children. Pediatric tourniquets should be used as well.

For all patients, phlebotomists must extract only the minimum volume, ensuring no duplicate requests and avoiding repeat collections.

Step 12. Apply Pressure over the Puncture Site with Clean Gauze

Improperly removing a needle can result in **hematoma**.

Technical Errors Leading to Hematoma Formation:

1. Forgetting to release the tourniquet before withdrawing the needle
2. Inadequate pressure applied to the site
3. Bending the patient's elbow over the site
4. Improper probing
5. Improper needle insertion technique
6. Using a large needle on a small vein
7. Puncturing the brachial artery

In geriatric patients, veins are less elastic and bruise more easily. Take care to use smaller needles.

In case a hematoma forms, immediately remove the needle and apply adequate pressure for two minutes or longer. You can advise the patient to use a cold compress for the next 24 hours, followed by a warm compress to reduce swelling.

Step 13. Discard Sharps

Step 14. Label Each Tube While the Patient Is Still in the Room

Observe the tubes for visible **hemolysis**. This is indicated by a pink or reddish tint on the plasma. Tests cannot be run on these specimens since the contents of the red blood cells have already contaminated the serum or plasma.

Preventable Errors Leading to Hemolysis

1. Using a 23-gauge needle, which has a bore that is too narrow
2. Improperly assembled devices
3. Pulling a syringe plunger too hard
4. Extraction on an area with hematoma
5. Shaking evacuated tubes
6. Tourniquet used for more than a minute
7. Alcohol still wet when venipuncture was performed
8. Probing improperly
9. Collecting from a sclerosed vein

Hemolysis can also occur during specimen processing. Rimming a clot, improper centrifugation, temperature extremes or improper pneumatic tube transport in unsuitable canisters contributes to hemolysis.

These can significantly affect laboratory results.

Troponin levels, liver enzymes, serum potassium, complete blood counts and lactate dehydrogenase assays rely on the specimen's integrity.

Other tests that are affected include FT4, coagulation assays, iron and haptoglobin, calcium and magnesium.

Step 15. Watch Out for Adverse Reactions

It is prudent to ask your patients, especially the elderly, about using blood thinners and herbal medications. This will indicate the need for more pressure.

If there is excess bleeding after applying five minutes of adequate pressure, you may need to ask your patients if they have been taking herbal medications. Bleeding is a common adverse effect of herbal medicine. It should be noted on the requisitions.

Common herbal medications that may affect coagulation tests and increase bleeding are celery, sweet clover, evening primrose oil, ginseng, garlic, ginger, vitamin E, coenzyme Q10, cat's claw, grapeseed oil, licorice, St. John's wort, ginkgo biloba, green tea, omega-3, turmeric.

It is not recommended to leave a patient who is still bleeding.

When bleeding is uncontrolled, especially in patients with a clotting disorder (von Willebrand disease or hemophilia) or on anticoagulants, blood continues to leak into the subcutaneous tissue. It can accumulate and cause a buildup of pressure. When this compresses a muscle, it is called **compartment syndrome**. This is a serious condition, causing painful inflammation that can compress a nerve. Always check the venipuncture site for bleeding and hematoma before applying bandages.

When you accidentally puncture the artery, noted by the unusually bright-red blood spurting into the tube, you must apply pressure for at least five minutes. Do not ask the patient to do this. Increase the time to 10 minutes if the patient is on anticoagulants. Failing to do so also results in compartment syndrome as well as nerve injuries.

Record on the requisition slip that the specimen is arterial blood since the reference ranges are different from tests on venous blood.

If a patient is allergic to adhesives, wrap gauze around their arm beforehand taping or use paper tape. When a patient has hirsute arms, do not use a bandage. You may use self-adhering bandages.

Do not bandage young children, particularly below two years old. They may ingest the bandages.

Instruct each patient to remove the bandage only after 15 minutes to **avoid infections**.

Step 16. Discard Used Supplies

Step 17. Thank the Patient

As you thank and leave the patients in the wards or hospital rooms, they may often ask you to change their bed positions or for a drink of water. This may not be in their best interests, such as with patients on a nothing-per-orem order in preparation for surgery. Politely let them know that you will inform their nurse of their requests.

Leave the room as you entered it. Remember to return the bed rails to avoid fall injuries.

Step 18. Deliver the Specimen

Instances When a Specimen Is Rejected

1. No labels or improper labels
2. Underfilled tubes
3. Using the wrong tubes
4. Hemolyzed samples
5. Lipemic samples
6. Presence of clots in an anticoagulated tube
7. Improper handling, such as not covering a light-sensitive specimen
8. Contaminated containers
9. Delayed transport
10. Using an expired tube
11. Specimen with no requisition form

Chapter 7: Dermal Puncture

Principles of Dermal Puncture

Dermal puncture refers to sampling blood from a capillary specimen. This is preferable for children (24 months old and younger) with lower blood volume and often no suitable superficial veins.

Instances When Adults Require a Dermal Puncture

- Burn patients
- Patients with extensive scarring
- Patients undergoing chemotherapy or frequent laboratory tests with reserved veins
- Elderly patients
- Patients with inaccessible veins (i.e., thrombosed, obesity)
- Patients on glucose monitoring

Instances When Dermal Puncture Is Unsuitable

- Patients with severe dehydration
- Patients with edematous fingers
- Tests requiring larger blood volumes (i.e., coagulation assays, ESR, blood culture)

Following correct dermal puncture techniques maintains the integrity of the test specimen.

Causes of Hemolysis on Dermal Punctures

- Milking or squeezing the site excessively
- Wet alcohol on the area
- Vigorously mixing the tubes

Newborn blood is inherently fragile and has an elevated red cell concentration. It is more prone to hemolysis.

Capillary blood is a mixture of oxygen-rich blood from the arterioles and oxygen-poor blood from the venules. However, the blood sample collected from capillary blood is a closer representation of an arterial than a venous sample.

Dermal puncture also collects some interstitial and intercellular fluid (fluids around and within the cells, respectively). Milking the site expresses these fluids and dilutes the sample.

The dermal puncture draws out a capillary sample. It contains higher glucose levels and lower potassium, calcium and protein levels than venous blood. Analytes from capillary blood may require a different set of **reference values**.

Be sure to make a note of when the dermal puncture was performed to alert the physicians as they interpret the test results.

Glucose and electrolyte levels are often serially determined. For better comparison, it is best not to switch between venipuncture and dermal punctures on the same patient.

Dermal Puncture Supplies

Dermal Puncture Devices

Dermal puncture devices are lancets with an automatically retractable safety feature. These devices contain a spring to control the puncture depth to a maximum of 2 mm. This depth avoids reaching the bone. For this reason, phlebotomists should never perform a puncture using uncontrolled surgical blades.

Separate devices are available for use on preterm neonates, newborns and older infants. Finger puncture devices are specially designed for use on toddlers, children and adults.

The volume of blood from a dermal puncture depends largely on the width of the puncture. This correlates with the number of capillaries severed. Several devices can vary puncture widths from pinpoint up to 2.5 mm.

Depending on the tests being ordered, you may need just a single drop of blood or a few milliliters in microcollection tubes.

Capillary Tube

Otherwise known as **microhematocrit tubes**, these are small containers that can hold about 50 to 70 microliters. These were designed to fit a hematocrit centrifuge and reader. The primary test they can run is a **hematocrit determination**.

These tubes come plain or heparinized. Plain tubes are used for transferring venipuncture specimens from lavender (EDTA) evacuated tubes, while heparinized tubes are used for dermal punctures.

Microcollection Tubes

These are miniature collection tubes colored to match the evacuated tubes but designed to collect capillary blood. They contain no vacuum and are used for dermal punctures. **BD Microtainers**® are manufactured with leak-proof caps, which are twisted and lifted off. These contain both minimum and maximum marks. Once filled, the caps are replaced and anticoagulated tubes are inverted for 5 to 10 inversions.

A **tube extender** is available to allow easy handling and adequate space for labels.

Other devices, such as **MiniCollect**®, **SAFE-T-FILL**® and **Microvette**®, incorporate a plastic capillary tube into the container. They also come with color-coded closures.

Amber-colored containers are available for photosensitive specimens.

Additional Supplies

Skin cleansers, gauze pads, a **sharps bin** and indelible **pens** are necessary.

A **glass slide** may be needed to prepare a blood smear.

Heel warmers, packets of sodium thiosulfate with glycerin, produce heat when the packet is squeezed and the contents are mixed. Keep a **towel** to wrap these packets when activating initially. A **warm washcloth** is a suitable alternative.

Dermal Puncture Procedure

Preparation

The dermal puncture begins with the requisition form. It should contain all the necessary information. Make a note that the specimen was collected by a dermal puncture.

You must prepare all the necessary equipment. Consider the volume of blood needed and the patient's age and condition before attempting to proceed.

Often, dermal punctures are performed in neonatal units or nurseries. These areas have established isolation protocols, such as handwashing and PPE. These must be duly observed to protect these patients.

Dermal punctures are often performed in the pediatric age group. Always remember to keep your supplies away from these patients' reach.

Identifying the Patient

The same procedures apply to identifying each patient. Verify the information on each requisition slip with the ID bands worn by the patient, not just placed above their beds or on their cribs.

Verbal identification of very young patients may be taken from their guardians. Note the informant's names on the requisition slip.

Meeting the Patient

You must approach pediatric patients in a friendly and confident manner. Explain the procedure to both patients and their guardians. Never promise that there will be no pain. Emphasize the need to remain still.

Allow guardians to leave the room if they prefer. If they choose to remain, ask for their assistance to comfort and hold the patient.

Very agitated children may need their legs and hands restrained or may be wrapped in a blanket or embraced by their guardians. Parents must consent to restrain the child. Properly document this on the chart.

Agitation and crying may affect white cell counts and blood glucose levels. Make a note of this event on the requisition form.

Positioning the Patient

For finger punctures: The patient is positioned either sitting or supine. Place the patient's nondominant hand on a firm surface. The palm is facing upward while the fingers are pointing down.

For heel punctures: The infant is supported on the back, with the heel positioned below the torso.

Site Selection

Consider the patient's age and weight when choosing the puncture site. The main concern is to avoid puncturing the bone and consequently introducing pathogens. This can lead to bone infections (**osteomyelitis**) or inflammation (**osteochondritis**).

Select a site that provides some distance from the skin and bone. Either the heel or the pads of the middle and ring fingers are suitable areas. Earlobe punctures are not recommended.

Avoid areas with poor circulation, such as calluses, scars, bruises, edema, infection and cyanosis.

Never repeat a puncture on a previous site. This can introduce pathogens and promote infections.

Secure the physician's permission before performing a finger puncture on the side of a recent mastectomy.

Heel Punctures

The heel is ideal for a dermal puncture in infants (less than 12 months old) because it provides more space between the skin and bone than their fingers.

Suitable areas for heel punctures are on the bottom of the heel, at either the medial or lateral surfaces. These areas provide the most space from the skin to the calcaneus bone. To locate these safe areas, trace a line from the middle of the big toe down to the heel. Alternately, trace from the fourth and fifth toes to the heel.

Do not attempt heel punctures on the back of the heel or the toes and arches. These areas are too close to other sensitive structures.

Finger Punctures

Finger punctures are ideal for adults and children over 12 months old.

Suitable areas for finger punctures are the pads (or the central areas) of the middle and ring fingers of the nondominant hand.

Avoid puncturing the tops and sides of the fingers.

Other fingers are not suitable. Thumbs may be callused. The index fingers contain more nerve endings. The little fingers have less tissue.

Warming the Sites

Warming the skin increases blood circulation. This eases the specimen collection. It is optimal for collecting multiple samples, capillary blood glucose sampling and cold and cyanotic areas.

Warm the site with a washcloth at 42° Celsius or use a heel warmer. The area is allowed to warm for about three to five minutes (but less than 10 minutes). This is effective in warming the area without affecting the test results.

Be very careful not to cause burns, especially in very young children.

Cleansing the Skin

Cleanse the site with 70% isopropyl alcohol. It must be allowed to dry before the procedure. Failing to do so may cause pain, rapid hemolysis and specimen contamination. This also causes collection difficulties since the admixture of blood and alcohol prevents the round blood drop from forming.

Povidone-iodine is not recommended in dermal punctures. It alters the test results for uric acid, bilirubin, phosphorus and potassium.

Puncturing the Skin

Hold the chosen puncture site firmly, but do not squeeze. Instead, apply gentle pressure to the area as you puncture. This increases the blood flow.

In heel punctures, the infant's heel is held between your nondominant thumb and index finger. Your index finger holds the foot arch while your thumb holds the bottom. Your other fingers wrap around the dorsal foot.

In finger punctures, the finger is held between your nondominant thumb and index finger. The patient's palm is facing upward while the fingers are pointing down.

Secure your selected puncture device. Take off the trigger lock if equipped. Firmly position the device on the site, taking care not to apply too much pressure. The device's blade is aligned across the grooves of the skin to create a perpendicular cut. This allows you to collect most of the blood, as it does not flow into these grooves.

Press on the device to release the lancet and puncture the skin. Briefly keep the pressure on the area before you remove the device. This avoids the skin's natural tendency to inhibit the blade from penetrating.

Removing the lancet prematurely causes an incomplete puncture. A common cause for the failure of dermal punctures is not holding the device firmly enough on the skin.

A new device must be used for every dermal puncture attempt.

Discard the Sharps

Dispose of used puncture devices in the appropriate sharps bin immediately.

Specimen Collection

Wipe off the initial drop with gauze. This avoids contamination from residual alcohol or tissue fluids. Do not milk the area. Blood should be allowed to flow freely into the microcollection tubes.

Gently applying and then releasing pressure about half an inch away from the area will allow for better blood flow.

The collecting devices should not touch the skin or scoop the blood. This can hemolyze the blood cells and contaminate the sample.

Capillary tubes draw blood through capillary action as the tip contacts the sample. The tube is positioned horizontally over the drop of blood until it fills. Moving the tip away from the blood prematurely causes air to collect in the tube and form bubbles. When the tubes have filled, they are covered with sealant clay or plastic closures.

Microcollection tubes are positioned at a downward angle, allowing the specimen to run down its side. The tips of these tubes are positioned beneath the drop of blood. You may need to tap these tubes to force the blood down the bottom. When it has filled, cover it with its colored cap. Additive tubes are inverted appropriately (see list below).

When taking multiple samples, it is crucial to move fast. Taking longer than two minutes causes microclots, which interfere with the test results.

Collect enough blood, as indicated by the marks on the tubes. Overfilling causes clots, while underfilling alters cell morphology.

When you are short on blood, a second puncture may be attempted with a new lancet. Do not add this new blood to an underfilled tube. This alters the test results.

Microtainer™ Color-Coded Caps

- **Lavender**
  Additive: Dipotassium EDTA
  Number of inversions: 10
  Specimen: Whole blood
  Use: Hematology assays

- **Green**
  Additive: Lithium heparin
  Number of inversions: 10
  Specimen: Plasma
  Use: Chemistry assays

- **Mint Green** (also comes in **amber** with mint-green caps)
  Additive: Lithium heparin and gel (plasma separator)
  Number of inversions: 10
  Specimen: Plasma
  Use: Chemistry assays

- **Gray**
  Additive: Sodium fluoride/EDTA
  Number of inversions: 10
  Specimen: Whole blood
  Use: Glucose tests

- **Gold** (also comes in **amber** with **gold** caps)
  Additive: Clot activator and serum separator gel
  Number of inversions: 5
  Specimen: Serum
  Use: Chemistry assays

- **Red**
  Additive: None
  Number of inversions: 0, none
  Specimen: Serum
  Use: Chemistry, immunoserology assays; blood banking

Order of Draw

Review the topic on hemostasis and coagulation. After the tissue is wounded, such as in a dermal puncture, platelets accumulate and aggregate. Considering this, tests to be used to study platelets should be collected first, before they can accumulate and alter the results. These include samples for blood smears, platelet counts and complete blood counts.

The order of draw is as follows:

- Capillary blood glucose
- Blood smear
- Lavender
- Heparinized tubes (green, mint green or amber with mint-green cap)
- Gray
- Serum tubes (gold or amber with gold cap)
- Red

Bandaging the Patient

After blood collection, use clean gauze to cover the area. Elevate the patient's hand or foot and place enough pressure to arrest the bleeding. Check that bleeding has ceased before covering the site with a bandage.

Instruct the patient to remove the bandage after 15 minutes.

Skip the bandage on young children (less than two years old).

Consider the sensitive skin of infants and the elderly before applying adhesive bandages.

Labeling

Label each specimen in front of the patient. Every tube should contain the same information as venipuncture tubes.

A label can be wrapped around a set of capillary tubes or the microcollection containers.

For transport, capillary tubes are kept in a larger tube to avoid exposure to the blood that has contaminated these tubes and to avoid breakage.

For microtainers, a tube extender may be available.

Completing the Procedure

Collect all used materials and used gloves and dispose of them in appropriate bins. Perform hand hygiene. Thank your patients and their guardians.

Observe standard precautions.

Observe priorities, such as STAT and timed specimens.

A log sheet documents the volume of blood drawn from each infant following every procedure. Document your dermal puncture to avoid iatrogenic anemia in these patients.

Only two attempts at dermal puncture are allowed for each patient.

Special Considerations During Dermal Puncture

Newborn Bilirubin

Bilirubin is a frequently requested assay on newborns. Often it is collected serially with timed intervals.

Certain conditions may increase bilirubin levels. Some are physiologic due to underdeveloped livers of preterm infants. Some may be pathologic, such as from ABO blood type incompatibility.

Determination of bilirubin levels is critical in managing neonates and preventing kernicterus (bilirubin accumulation in the brain). This is potentially life-threatening.

Bilirubin is photosensitive and destroyed by light exposure. These specimens must be collected in amber containers or protected from exposure to light pre- and post-collection.

Jaundiced infants (yellowish skin and eyes from increased bilirubin) are treated by being placed under an ultraviolet lamp. You must remember to turn this off throughout the dermal puncture process.

It is important to follow the indicated timing on bilirubin requisitions. This allows the physician to assess the progression of jaundice.

Chapter 8: Newborn Screening

Tests for inborn errors of metabolism and certain inherited conditions are available for neonates. Detecting these conditions early may prevent complications, especially physical and mental impairments and early death.

Current laboratory assays may detect as many as 50 of these conditions. The required specific screening varies with each state.

Regardless, all states include screening for these four conditions:

Cystic fibrosis is a rare genetic condition from a mutation that affects chloride transport at the cellular level. This causes the overproduction of mucous that eventually blocks the bronchioles.

Phenylketonuria is is a congenital metabolic disorder characterized by the body's inability to metabolize the amino acid phenylalanine. Without the necessary enzyme to convert phenylalanine into tyrosine, the buildup of phenylalanine can disrupt brain development. However, damage can be prevented through a specific diet that limits phenylalanine intake.

Galactosemia is due to the lack of an enzyme that normally metabolizes galactose, which is found in milk. This accumulates in the blood and causes problems in multiple organs, such as the liver, brain and kidneys. The damage is prevented by placing these infants on a lactose-free and galactose-free diet.

Congenital hypothyroidism is an inborn deficiency from an underdeveloped thyroid. Undetected and untreated, it can lead to delayed growth and brain retardation (traditionally described as cretinism). Treatment involves supplementation with thyroid hormones.

Early detection of these conditions is crucial because the damage (often permanent) is caused by the accumulation of certain metabolites (which can be prevented).

Screening for these conditions is performed on a dermal puncture sample taken between 24 and 48 hours after delivery.

Newborn Screening Procedure

When asked to perform this procedure, you will receive a specimen card or a **Guthrie card**. This special filter paper is attached to a form bearing the neonate's information (like a requisition form).

The blood from the heel puncture is blotted on an area marked by circles on the Guthrie card. You must avoid contaminating this area with other chemicals or even your fingerprints.

Use only one drop of blood on each circle and apply each to the same side. Do not touch the paper to the infant's heel. An adequate sample is also visible on the back side of the card.

Each circle must be adequately filled. If one was incorrectly filled, use a new circle to avoid layering.

After filling all the circles, air-dry the card horizontally. Shield it from direct sunlight.

After at least three hours, it may be sealed in its designated envelope to be mailed to the testing laboratory.

A Newborn Screening Card May Be Rejected Due To:

- An **insufficient sample** from removing the paper prematurely before the blood had time to fill the circle or soak through or from touching the paper with gloves
- A **scratched specimen** from the use of a capillary pipette to apply the blood
- **Inadequately drying** the sample
- **Oversaturation** with excess blood from the use of devices
- **Diluted or contaminated samples** from milking the site
- **Serum rings** from contamination with wet alcohol or other substances, improper drying or use of pipettes
- **Clotting** from the application of several drops of blood on one circle or applying the blood to both sides of the card

Chapter 9: Peripheral Blood Smears

A blood smear is a film of blood on a glass slide. This allows the cells to be viewed under a microscope for a white cell differential count, special stains and manual reticulocyte counts.

You may be requested to prepare a peripheral blood smear from either a venipuncture or a dermal puncture.

Collecting the Blood Smear Sample

For dermal punctures, collection of the blood smear sample takes priority over any other tubes. This is to avoid collecting blood with platelet clumps.

For venipunctures, the smear is prepared from blood collected in EDTA tubes. This should be prepared within the hour of collection. Prolonged exposure to EDTA causes cells to appear distorted. The tube is mixed for two minutes. Then a sample is collected with a plain capillary tube. Transfer one drop of blood on a glass slide. You can prepare the smear manually or with the use of an automated instrument.

Preparing a Thin Blood Smear

Manually preparing a smear requires much practice.

After collecting the blood, a drop of it (1 to 2 mm in diameter) is placed on the center of a glass slide, either by a capillary tube (in venipuncture) or from the dermal puncture. Take a clean, smooth-edged slide to use as the spreader slide. At a 30° or 40° angle, collect the blood toward the back of the spreader slide; allow it to spread evenly. Then lightly push it forward, maintaining the angle, continuously for the entire slide length.

A properly prepared smear has a smooth film covering about two-thirds of the slide without any creases or holes. It ends smoothly as a **feathered edge.** This area ensures that the cells are spread in a single even layer. The feathered edge is the area viewed under the microscope to ensure the reader is looking at a sample representative of the patient's blood.

Allow the slide to air-dry while you prepare another smear.

Wear your gloves throughout the procedure. The specimen is potentially infectious until it has been fixed in alcohol.

Write the labels with a pencil on the frosted end of the slide. Keep the smears in a transport container. Discard the spreader slides.

Technical Errors Encountered in the Preparation of Blood Smears

- Unevenly distributed blood due to excess pressure or noncontinuous movement of the spreader slide or from dried blood due to delay in preparing the smear
- Holes due to dirt or glove powder
- Failure to create a feathered edge by abruptly ceasing the spreader slide
- Streaks on the feathered edge caused by a chipped spreader slide or from dried blood due to a delay in preparing the smear
- Using an angle of more than 40° or a large drop of blood, creating a smear that is too thick and short
- Using an angle less than 30° or pushing the spreader slide too slowly, creating a smear that is too thin and long

Blood Smears for Malaria

Both thick and thin blood smears are used to detect malarial parasites *(Plasmodium sp.)* inside the erythrocytes. This disease causes an episodic fever corresponding to the proliferation of these parasites within the erythrocytes. The specimen may be collected at intervals of 8 to 12 hours for two to three days.

Thin smears are used to identify parasites based on their morphologic characteristics.

Thick smears prepare a concentrated sample to find and detect these parasites.

Preparing a Thick Blood Smear

Place a large drop of blood on the center of the slide. Spread the sample into a circle with an applicator stick or another glass slide. Air-dry the smear for at least two hours before staining.

Chapter 10: Blood Culture

Collection of blood culture specimens is one of your most challenging duties as a phlebotomist.

Bacteremia is the presence of bacteria in the bloodstream. Sepsis is the clinical term used when the patient has a systemic inflammation (such as fever and increased heart rate or increased white cell counts), along with bacteremia.

Blood culture results report the growth or absence of bacteria after every 24 hours. If bacteria are able to grow, further chemical and microscopic analyses are done to identify the genus and species.

Antibiotic susceptibility is also performed to identify which antibiotic can be used against these bacteria and which antibiotic they can resist.

Timing of Blood Culture Collection

Physicians may request the specimen as either STAT or timed collection.

Blood culture is usually collected as two sets of blood taken 30 minutes or one hour apart.

Some physicians may request the cultures be collected just before the height of the fever (based on the patterns in the temperature charts) to collect the most concentration of pathogens.

Certain life-threatening conditions, such as bacterial meningitis, may require empiric antibiotics to be started immediately. The patient is often given an antibiotic that covers the most common causative agents. A blood culture may be requested as STAT at the emergency department just before the antibiotics are given. In this case, you will simultaneously draw both blood culture sets from different venipuncture sites.

These specimens must be labeled with the site and order of collection (i.e., left arm antecubital vein #1).

Aseptic Technique

Proper adherence to aseptic techniques is crucial. Human skin is normally covered in normal bacterial flora. Any contamination can introduce these bacteria into the sample and cause erroneous results.

Collection Equipment

Blood Culture Collection Containers

Blood culture bottles contain culture media (a mixture of nutrients required to grow bacteria) and an anticoagulant (sodium polyanethole sulfonate).

Alternatively, a **sterile yellow (SPS) evacuated tube** may be used to collect the sample. This tube contains the same anticoagulant. The blood is then inoculated onto appropriate culture media in the laboratory.

When using a winged (butterfly) collection system, use one with a **Leuer adapter** and a transfer device so blood flows continuously from the puncture site into the culture bottles without contamination.

When using a syringe system, ensure adherence to aseptic techniques. Always use a sterile transfer device to transfer the specimen into the culture bottles. Do not inoculate the syringe into the culture bottles. This can increase your exposure to blood-borne pathogens.

Special blood culture bottles are available when it is necessary to take a blood culture sample from patients who are already taking antibiotics. These may contain resins (**antimicrobial removal devices**) or activated charcoal (**fastidious antimicrobial neutralization**), which are designed to inactivate antibiotics.

Only trained staff can collect specimens from vascular access devices (such as IV catheters or ports). However, collecting from VADs is associated with more contamination than venipuncture.

The **Steripath ISDD®** is a closed system collection designed to prevent contamination from equipment and skin flora by mechanically diverting the first 1.5 to 2 milliliters of blood into a separate chamber. This system substantially reduces contamination to only 0.2%.

Blood Culture Anticoagulants

Anticoagulation is necessary to prevent trapping microbes in clots that may remain undetected. Tubes must be inverted after blood collection. **Sodium polyanethole sulfonate** is the only suitable anticoagulant for blood cultures because it allows bacteria to grow.

Blood Culture Procedure

The collection begins with obtaining a complete requisition form. You must prepare all the necessary equipment and plan to perform two venipunctures for each of the two specimens. Consider the volume of blood needed as well as the age and condition of patients and their veins.

Identifying the Patient

Verify the information on each requisition form with the ID bands worn by the patient. Whenever possible, always ask for verbal identification. Two identifiers are required.

Meeting the Patient

Explain the procedure to the patient. Emphasize that the specimen needs to be collected from two separate punctures to avoid contamination.

Verify allergies since you will be cleansing the site with multiple cleansers.

Position the Patient and Identify the Site

Refer to the routine venipuncture procedure in chapter 5.

Cleanse the Site

The main difference between venipunctures and blood culture collection lies in skin preparation. Extensive skin preparation in blood culture collection ensures the least amount of contamination.

Available skin cleansers are 2% tinctures of iodine, povidone-iodine, 70% isopropyl alcohol and chlorhexidine gluconates. These are all comparably effective in clearing bacteria off the skin.

Two-Step Method. This uses 70% isopropyl alcohol for one minute, followed by an iodine-containing cleanser for another minute. The site is scrubbed in a circular motion from the center, progressing outward three to four inches. Allow at least 30 seconds for the cleansers to dry before the venipuncture.

Iodine is possibly irritating and may be absorbed from the skin. After the procedure, wipe off the remaining iodine with alcohol swabs.

One-Step Method. ChloraPrep, a commercially prepared mixture of chlorhexidine gluconate and alcohol, is available as a swab. This method has been adopted by many facilities, especially for patients with iodine sensitivity. Using a ChloraPrep swab, scrub the site. Allow at least 30 seconds for the cleansers to dry before proceeding.

Chlorhexidine gluconate is not suitable for use on infants below two months old. It is highly irritating to their sensitive skin and may cause chemical burns.

When preparing equipment, the rubber stoppers of each blood culture bottle must also be cleansed with 70% alcohol after removing the plastic caps. Leave the alcohol pad to cover these bottles while you perform the venipuncture. Remove the pad only when ready to inoculate the specimen into the bottles.

Do not use iodine to cleanse the rubber stoppers. It can contaminate the specimen or deteriorate the rubber.

Specimen Collection

Proceed with the venipuncture as with other routine punctures.

When the specimen has been collected in a syringe, the anaerobic bottle (red blood culture bottle) is inoculated first. This prevents exposure to air, which can destroy anaerobic bacteria.

When a winged collection system is used, blood is collected in the aerobic bottle first. This ensures the air present in the tubing does not contaminate the anaerobic bottle.

Blood Culture Volume Requirements

Pediatric bottles are available for use on children. The volume of blood collected is computed based on the child's weight.

A sufficient sample is 1 mL for every 5 kilograms or 1 mL for every 10 lbs.

From children weighing over 45 kg, collect as much as an adult. From an infant weighing less than 5 kg, collect only 1 ml in only one bottle.

The ratio of blood to the culture medium is 1:10. Proper volumes must be collected to ensure the correct ratio. In adults, 8 to 10 mL of blood is collected per blood culture bottle. From pediatric patients, only 1 to 3 mL of blood is collected per pediatric bottle.

Chapter 11: Special Handling Requirements

Warming

A **cold agglutinin** is an autoantibody produced after cells encounter Mycoplasma pneumonia, the causative agent for walking pneumonia. Cold agglutinins may also be present in patients with autoimmune hemolytic anemia.

Cold agglutinins react with erythrocytes when subjected to temperatures lower than normal body temperature. Because the assay is run on serum samples, it is important to keep the blood warm until serum is collected. This ensures that cold agglutinins are present in the sample and have not attached to the erythrocytes.

The tubes should be free of additives and prewarmed at 37° C for 30 minutes. Transport the tube back to the laboratory in a warm container, with portable heat blocks or in your tightly clenched fist. The tubes may be kept in an incubator at 37° C until they are centrifuged and tested.

The same collection and handling procedure applies to **cryofibrinogen** and **cryoglobulin.**

Chilling

Keeping specimens chilled prevents the deterioration of sensitive analytes that may otherwise be metabolized in the blood at normal temperatures.

This is done by preparing a container with crushed ice or a uniform ice block to transport the specimen in. It is important to ensure that chilling occurs uniformly and that no part of the sample freezes. Freezing causes hemolysis.

Tests for acetone, arterial blood gases, pyruvate, lactic acid and ammonia require chilling. Hormone assays for ACTH, PTH, catecholamines and glucagon may also require chilling.

Chilling is not required for arterial blood gas specimens collected in a plastic syringe and analyzed in 30 minutes.

Chilling is not suitable for testing some analytes. Potassium increases in a chilled tube. Electrolyte tests must be collected separately when drawing blood with chilling requirements.

Factor VII may be activated in lower temperatures. Chilling is not recommended for testing prothrombin time and INR.

Protect from Light

Photosensitive analytes deteriorate upon exposure to light or ultraviolet radiation. These specimens may be wrapped in aluminum foil or collected in amber-colored tubes.

Photosensitive analytes include bilirubin, vitamin A, porphyrins, folate, niacin (vitamin B6) and cyanocobalamin (vitamin B12).

Chain-of-Custody Guidelines

You may be asked to collect forensic samples for use in legal proceedings. These are often tests for blood levels of drugs and alcohol or DNA samples. Follow the policies with extreme care.

Specimen handling is documented extensively on the **chain-of-custody form.** It starts with identifying the patient and collecting the specimen, witnessed by an officer of the law and continues until the laboratory results are reported.

Additional patient identifiers may be required, such as fingerprints or heel prints (in paternity cases).

Each person involved in the chain of custody must document their name and the date and time they handled the specimen.

The information is collected on special forms, which require appropriate seals.

Blood Alcohol Collection

When collecting samples for blood alcohol levels, the site is cleansed with solutions other than 70% isopropyl alcohol. This may be soap and water or benzalkonium (Zephiran) chloride.

Alcohol is a volatile substance and may escape into the surrounding air. Gray tubes (with sodium fluoride) must be filled until the vacuum is exhausted. They must remain covered until testing.

Underfilling and uncapping the tubes allow alcohol to escape into the surrounding air, resulting in falsely low blood alcohol levels.

Molecular Testing

This field was designed for use in DNA testing. It was originally for forensic and paternity purposes. It has now expanded to identify viral organisms (HIV, HCV), hematologic conditions and genetic disorders.

Specimens collected depend on the test requested.

Paternity testing samples are commonly collected in yellow (acid citrate dextrose) tubes. Other tests may be collected in EDTA-containing tubes or sodium citrate anticoagulated tubes.

Chapter 12: Blood Donation

Phlebotomists may be assigned to blood collection centers.

Your tasks at these blood collection centers include the initial assessment of donors and extend throughout the procedure until the donor is safely dismissed from the blood collection center.

Donor Screening

Every volunteer undergoes a thorough interview and physical examination to ensure that the procedure will not cause them any harm and that their blood will not be harmful to others.

The interview is extensive and includes some sensitive questions. It should be held in a private area. Volunteers are encouraged to be truthful, as their blood could pose a health risk to recipients. The questions cover medical history, current medication use, smoking and drinking habits and history of drug abuse, sexually transmitted diseases or exposure to blood-borne pathogens.

Eligibility Criteria for Blood Donation

- At least 17 years old; some states allow 16-year-olds to donate with consent from their parents or guardians
- At least 110 pounds or 50 kg in weight
- Afebrile (body temperature must not exceed 99.5°F)
- Blood pressure at least 90/50 but below 180/100 mmHg
- Pulse rate within the normal range of 50 to 100 bpm
- Hemoglobin at least 12.5 g/dL
- Without skin lesions; track marks on the forearms may indicate IV drug use
- At least eight weeks since the last blood donation

Volunteers may continue to take antihypertensive medications, oral contraceptive pills, hormone replacement therapy and/or insulin.

Volunteers who have bleeding conditions or take blood thinners are deferred from donating. Donation of whole blood is allowable while on aspirin. Aspirin must be discontinued for two days before donation by platelet apheresis.

Volunteers taking antibiotics for infections must wait until they have taken the last pill of a full course before being eligible.

Recent vaccinations are allowed, but at least four weeks should pass after immunization with live vaccines (Zostavax for shingles; MMR; varicella) and at least two weeks for the live COVID-19 vaccine, rubeola oral polio vaccine and yellow fever vaccine.

At least 21 days should pass after immunization for hepatitis B (primary course).

Donor screening also involves ABO and Rh blood type testing. Donor blood is screened for the following:

- Human immunodeficiency virus
- Hepatitis B and C
- Human T-lymphotropic virus
- West Nile virus
- *Trypanosoma cruzi*
- *Treponema pallidum*

Volunteers must pass this screen before they can donate their blood. This ensures that this blood is safe for recipients.

Donors are also given a private opportunity to indicate whether they would deny permission to use their blood for transfusion. This may be done by providing a sealed form with tick boxes indicating "use" or "do not use." The seal is opened only after the blood unit has been collected. Alternatively, donors may be given two labels indicating "use" or "do not use," which they can attach to the collected unit.

Donor Identification

Donors are asked to present valid ID bearing their full name, birth date, address, contact information and sex. This may vary per facility.

The donor registry may be verified to see whether a volunteer was previously deferred (or disqualified) from blood donation.

Securing an Informed Consent

The procedure should be explained thoroughly, along with its risks. The donors are asked to sign a document expressing their consent for the venipuncture and testing.

Donor Blood Collection

A blood unit comes as a sterile closed-system bag with tubings connected to a sterile needle. A large-gauge needle (16- or 17-gauge) is necessary to prevent hemolysis and allow large volumes to be collected. A thin-walled needle is available, which provides a large bore in a diameter that does not cause too much discomfort. The blood bags are placed lower than the arm. This allows them to fill by gravity. They may be placed on a mixing device that automatically stops when the desired volume has been collected. When the collection is complete, a hemostat is attached to the tubing to stop the blood flow into the blood bags.

The blood bag contains **citrate-phosphate-dextrose** or **citrate-phosphate-dextrose-adenine**. These additives preserve the blood and prevent clots. The unit is designed to collect 405 to 495 milliliters of blood. This can be processed to obtain the necessary blood components, such as packed red cells, platelets and plasma proteins.

Donors need to have adequately large antecubital veins to accommodate the large-gauge needles.

Employing aseptic techniques is essential to prevent contamination of the blood units. Adequate skin cleansing requires two steps. First, by soap and water or a detergent scrub, then by application of iodine or chlorhexidine gluconate. Allow at least 30 seconds for the cleansers to dry before proceeding.

The venipuncture is performed in the usual manner. Donors are encouraged to pump their fist to allow a faster blood flow.

Donor Apheresis Collection

Apheresis is a method of collecting a specified blood component.

The desired blood component is collected while the volunteer is still connected to the machine. The apheresis device holds a centrifuge that separates whole blood into its components through density. The density of blood components in decreasing order are red cells, white cells, platelets and plasma.

A specially trained phlebotomist directs the required blood component into the blood bag unit. The rest of the blood is returned to the donor without leaving the sterile chambers of the machine.

Autologous Donation

Patients who need elective surgery may preemptively donate a unit of their blood to be transfused during or after their operation. An autologous donation avoids transfusion reactions and exposure to bloodborne pathogens.

If multiple blood units are required, a patient may donate every three days, with the physician's approval and adequate hemoglobin level.

These autologous units are reserved solely for their donor.

Post-Donation Care

Once the blood bag has filled, use the hemostat to clamp the tubing. The needle is then removed. Firm pressure should be applied to the site while the donor's arm is elevated.

During this time, dispose of the needle appropriately and transfer blood from the tubing into the appropriate tubes for testing. Label each unit appropriately.

Confirm that the bleeding has stopped before applying a sterile gauze and bandaging the site. Instruct the donors to remove these after 4 hours.

Always observe the donors for any signs of nausea, dizziness or fainting until after bandaging them. Manage complications as described in Chapter 6.

Allow donors to have some juice or snacks before leaving the blood collection center. They should be instructed to drink plenty of fluids for the rest of the day and avoid strenuous activities or heavy lifting.

They should be told that they might feel nauseous or dizzy during the next 24 hours; if this happens, they should lie down or rest for a few minutes until they feel better.

Chapter 13: Other Duties of a Phlebotomist

Aside from blood collection, phlebotomists may be tasked to perform additional duties related to other specimens.

Depending on your facility, you may be asked to do any or all of the following:

- Instruct patients on collecting specimens for urinalysis, fecalysis or semen analysis.
- Collect throat or nasopharyngeal swabs.
- Collect sweat for electrolyte analysis.
- Assist oncologists or hematologists in performing bone marrow aspiration
- Transport and receive these specimens
- Perform blood donor interviews, screening, collection and processing

Patient Instructions for Urine Collection

Random Urine

This refers to samples collected without regard for timing. The patient is handed a specimen cup and directed to the toilet. This sample may be used for routine urinalysis.

First Morning Urine

This is preferred because it concentrates the analytes. It may be requested to confirm the results of random samples.

Patients are given a specimen cup to fill with urine during their first void in the morning. They are instructed to submit this within 2 hours.

24-Hour Sample

These timed samples provide a quantitative measure of urine analytes. Patients are given a large container with a preservative. These may be caustic. Patients should be advised accordingly.

Patients should be instructed on the importance of collecting all their urine into the container for the accuracy of the results.

Clean-Catch Midstream Sample

This is ideal for urine cultures. It avoids collecting contaminant organisms and cells from the external genitalia and the first and last parts of the urinary stream.

Patients are given sterile specimen cups and towelettes moistened with a mild antiseptic. They are directed to sanitize their hands first. They should be reminded not to touch the inside of these cups.

Instructions for cleansing genitalia: Women should hold their skin folds apart, while uncircumcised men are asked to retract their foreskin. They should wipe with the towelettes provided.

They are asked to first void into the toilet, then catch the middle stream of urine into the container without touching it on their skin. They can finish voiding into the toilet.

These samples should be delivered to the microbiology department right away.

Catheter Sample

For bacterial cultures, a sterile sample is required. Bedridden patients, infants and other patients may have conditions that make them unable to void. The urine specimen is collected by passing a sterile catheter into the patient's urethra under aseptic conditions. This is collected only by trained personnel.

You might be asked to transport the sample to the laboratory.

Suprapubic Aspiration

This is collected by trained personnel who insert a needle through the skin into the bladder. This is to ensure an uncontaminated sample for bacteriologic or cytologic examination, more often from infants or small children.

Your task might be to transport the sample to the laboratory.

Pediatric Sample

Urine from small children may be collected in a collection bag with hypoallergenic adhesives attached to their cleansed genital area. The diaper is then placed over the bag. When an adequate volume has been collected, the bag is labeled and transported to the laboratory.

Urine Drug Test

A drug test may be part of a forensic investigation or carry some legal implications. These tests require a clear **chain of custody** to ensure no tampering.

Patient ID requires a photo ID and may require fingerprints.

To ensure that specimen tampering cannot happen, patients are asked to deposit belongings, coats, purses and bags in lockers outside the drug testing area.

Drug-testing toilets have a blueing agent added to the reservoir. There should be no available water source in the area.

A **witnessed sample** may be required in certain situations. A same-sex staff observes patients as they collect 30 to 45 ml of urine.

The patient should hand the sample to the collector immediately. Within four minutes, the temperature of the sample is checked. If it is below 32.5° C or above 37.7° C, the collector is alerted to possible contamination. Inform the patient's supervisor or employers and collect a second sample.

The collector inspects the sample. Derangements in urine color, pH and specific gravity suggest contamination. Tampering is indicated by a pH above 9. Dilution lowers the specific gravity to <1.005.

If the specimen is adequate, the collector attaches the labels to the container in front of the patient. They are asked to affix initials on the specimen containers.

A completed chain-of-custody form, signed by the patient, collectors and any other handlers, is required for these tests.

Patient Instructions for Stool Collection

Random Stool Specimen

Random stool samples may be requested for the detection of ova and parasites and for fecal microscopy to analyze cells, fats and occult blood tests. Containers may be screw-capped cups, like those for urine or a wax-coated cardboard container. They may contain preservatives to allow the sample to be stored at room temperature.

A kit for occult blood testing contains filter paper impregnated with reagents.

72-Hour Timed Stool Specimen

A 72-hour timed specimen may be ordered for quantitative testing of stool fats.

A large container is kept in the laboratory. This is used to collect urine from the patient's bedpan or disposable containers. The patients are instructed to avoid contaminating the specimen with urine or water. The specimen should be refrigerated if a delay is expected before the sample can be sent to the laboratory.

Patient Instructions for Semen Collection

A semen sample may be analyzed to evaluate infertility and vasectomy and for forensic investigations.

Patients are instructed to refrain from sexual activity for three days but not more than five days.

Ideally, they are asked to come to the laboratory to collect the sample in a sterile cup. Condoms are not suitable since they may contain spermicides.

If patients prefer to collect the sample at home, instruct them to keep the sample warm (37° Celsius). It should be brought to the laboratory within an hour of collection.

Instruct patients to take note of the time of collection. When you receive the sample, record both the time of sample collection and the time it arrived. The life span of spermatozoa and liquefaction time are time-bound parameters of semen analysis.

Non-Blood Specimen Collections

Throat Swabs

You may be requested to collect a throat swab, especially from children, to detect streptococcal infections on culture or point-of-care tests.

To collect a sample, have patients tilt their head and open their mouth. Maintain an aseptic technique as you uncap the tube and take the swab. With a tongue depressor, gently lower the patient's tongue. Asking them to say "Ahhh" can also aid with the collection.

Direct the swab straight to the back of the throat. Be sure to swab areas with inflammation or ulceration. Do not touch the cheeks, teeth or lips throughout this process.

Return the sterile swab to its tube, replace the cap and label accordingly.

Some test kits contain an ampule with transport media for the bacteria to remain alive. This needs to be crushed to release the contents to contact the swab.

The specimen should be sent to the microbiology department immediately.

Nasopharyngeal Swabs

Nasopharyngeal swabs were previously requested from infants for the detection of respiratory syncytial viruses, influenza viruses and Bordetella pertussis.

Nowadays, it is mainly indicated for molecular testing for SARS-CoV-2, the virus responsible for COVID-19.

A sterile mini-tip swab is inserted gently through the nostril into the nasopharynx. It is gently rotated and removed. For COVID-19 point-of-care tests, some manufacturers require repeating the procedure on the second nostril.

The swab is immersed and vigorously mixed in a saline transport medium. The excess liquid should be squeezed out of the swab before disposing of it.

The tube is labeled accordingly and transported on an ice slurry to the laboratory.

Assisting Physicians with Specimen Collection

Bone Marrow Aspiration

You may be requested to assist in collecting bone marrow for hematological analysis.

The oncologist or hematologist uses a thick **Jamshidi needle** to take a sample of the patient's bone marrow from their iliac crest.

You should prepare the materials and hand these in the correct order to the physician.

The physician aspirates liquid marrow into the syringe, then collects the bone core.

Prepare three or four slides for the core biopsy. The physician hands you the sample, which you will place on a sterile gauze. Use the slides to touch the samples gently, about three times each, to make an imprint. Transport the slides in a container of formalin.

Dispense three or four drops of bone marrow from the syringe on an angled slide supported by a Petri dish. These are used to make six to eight thin smears.

Collect 1 to 2 ml of bone marrow in EDTA and heparin-containing tubes. Invert these tubes.

The remaining bone marrow is allowed to clot within the syringe. The clotted marrow is transferred to another container of formalin.

Label all slides, tubes and formalin bottles accordingly. Include the dates and time of collection, the bone marrow site and your initials on the labels.

Deliver the specimen to histology for analysis. Their slides are sent to hematology for staining and microscopy.

Handling and Transporting Non-Blood Specimen

In the laboratory, you may also be assigned to transport, handle and receive specimens other than the blood you collected.

Along with specimens for urinalysis and fecalysis, you may be asked to handle cerebrospinal fluid and other fluids from the synovium, pleura and peritoneum, as well as hair and other tissues.

Most of these are collected in an invasive manner. These must be handled carefully and transported to the laboratory with utmost priority.

A pneumatic tube system is available in many hospitals to facilitate the delivery of specimens from the wards to the laboratory. Tubes must be properly cushioned and kept in leakproof biohazard containers.

Specimens collected through invasive means must be transported only by hand. This avoids any untoward incidents from a pneumatic tube transit.

These specimens must be received with their accompanying requisition forms and proper labels on the container itself. Make sure the labels are not written on the lids. This avoids mixing up specimens when the lids are opened.

When delivering these to their respective departments, inform the personnel about them. When there are none available, such as during late shifts, you should consult the procedural manual for specific specimen storage and handling requirements.

Amniotic Fluid

The unborn fetus lies within the amniotic fluid. Physicians may aspirate a sample of this through amniocentesis around the second trimester of pregnancy to investigate hemolytic disease or genetic disease or to ascertain fetal lung maturity.

From the amniotic fluid, alpha-fetoprotein levels and bilirubin levels are quantified to investigate fetal development.

Specimen handling requirements vary per test. You must refer to your facility's procedural manuals for specimen handling requirements.

Tissue Samples

These are routinely received following excision or biopsy. They are often fixed in a preservative solution or delivered immediately to the histology department.

Cerebrospinal Fluid (CSF)

This fluid surrounds the cranial and spinal cord meninges, which serve to cushion these sensitive areas, supply nutrients and remove metabolic waste.

Collection of CSF is done by a physician through a **lumbar puncture procedure**.

A needle is inserted between the L3, L4 and L5 lumbar vertebrae. It is possible to collect the fluid in these areas without damaging the spinal cord.

The samples are used to investigate the organisms responsible for meningitis and other neurological pathologies.

The fluid is collected in three sterile tubes labeled according to the collection order.

The first tube is intended for chemistry and immunoserology assays. This often contains cells or microorganisms obtained from the puncture procedure, not normally found in the CSF. The second tube is for microbiology, and the third is for hematology and cytology.

When a fourth tube is collected, the tubes are labeled differently. The first and last tubes are sent to hematology. This allows a comparison to determine contamination with red cells, especially after a traumatic collection. The second tube is for chemistry and immunoserology, while the third tube is for microbiology.

These tests are always regarded as STAT because cells begin deteriorating within the first hour.

The tubes for chemistry and immunology may be refrigerated. Tubes for microbiology and hematology are kept at room temperature since fastidious microorganisms (such as Neisseria meningitides) cannot survive at lower temperatures.

Synovial Fluid

This is also known as joint fluid, which acts as a lubricant during movement. Its normal appearance is clear and colorless to pale or straw-colored.

During inflammatory states (such as arthritis), the volume of fluids in the affected joint increases. A physician aspirates the fluid through a needle, and the samples may be analyzed according to the desired tests.

Heparin-containing tubes are used for Gram stain and microbiologic culture. Either EDTA- or heparin-containing tubes are used for cell count and identification of crystals. Sodium fluoride-containing gray tubes are used for synovial fluid glucose tests. A plain sterile tube is used for other tests.

Serous Fluid

This is the collective term used to refer to the fluid found within the space created by the parietal and visceral membranes of organ cavities.

Types of Serous Fluids

SEROUS FLUID	LOCATION	INCREASED IN
Pleural	Lungs	Tuberculosis, lung infections, tumors
Pericardial	Heart	Heart failure, pericarditis
Peritoneal	Abdominal cavity	Hypoproteinemia, lymphatic obstruction

An increase in the pleural and pericardial fluid may be referred to clinically as pleural and pericardial effusion, respectively. An increase in the peritoneal fluid is also known as ascites.

Serous fluid specimens are often collected in tubes corresponding to the ones used for blood samples for similar tests.

Heparin-containing tubes are used for microbiology, cytology and chemistry. EDTA-containing tubes are used for cell and differential count.

Hair

Chronic drug, metals, toxins and alcohol intake deposits certain metabolites in the hair strands. Hair may also be used as a DNA sample for paternity tests. It is easy to collect and difficult to compromise.

Gastric Fluid

These are a series of specimens collected at timed intervals to investigate stomach acid production.

The first sample is collected through a gastric tube; then the patient is given histamine (to stimulate gastric acid production). Subsequent samples are collected at intervals. Labels should contain the time of collection.

A blood gastrin level test may be ordered. In this case, a venipuncture may be done concurrently.

Sputum

This refers to the mucus produced by the respiratory tract. It is increased during inflammatory states. Sputum tests are to investigate the causative agents in suspected tuberculosis and pneumonia.

A first-morning sample is ideal to ensure a large enough collection. Patients are instructed to collect the samples before a meal and without smoking.

Moments before the expectoration of sputum, have the patient gargle with water (but do not swallow) to obtain a sample with the least contamination.

Sputum samples are delivered to the laboratory immediately and kept at room temperature.

Take airborne precautions when handling these samples. Always wear a mask.

Buccal Swabs

These are obtained by rubbing the cheek with a sterile cotton swab for about 20 seconds to collect cells for DNA testing. When collected for legal purposes, these may require a strict chain-of-custody protocol.

Saliva

Salivary drug and alcohol levels can be determined immediately and are difficult to compromise. Certain point-of-care test kits use saliva samples.

It is also a less invasive test for the detection of HIV antibodies.

Breath

C-urea breath test

Helicobacter pylori bacteria colonize the stomach. This can lead to peptic and duodenal ulcers as well as chronic inflammation. It may be detected indirectly through the carbon dioxide content from a breath sample.

The procedure is as follows:

1. The patient breathes into a balloon device to collect a baseline sample.
2. The patient ingests C-urea (a carbon isotope that is not radioactive).
3. The patient breathes into another balloon device.

H. pylori produces **urease**, which degrades urea. During this process, carbon dioxide is released and may be captured in the balloon.

The levels of exhaled carbon dioxide from both balloons are compared. An increase in the second sample indicates infection with *H. pylori.*

Hydrogen Breath Test

This test is requested to investigate **malabsorption**. This requires a 12-hour fast.

The procedure is as follows:

1. The patient breathes into a balloon device to measure a baseline hydrogen level.
2. The patient ingests lactose.
3. The patient breathes into the balloon device, and the hydrogen level is serially measured every 15 minutes over 3 to 5 hours.

Increasing levels indicate malabsorption or indigestion of lactose in the gastrointestinal tract. This may aid in diagnosing lactose intolerance, small intestine bacterial overgrowth or dumping syndromes.

Alcohol Breath Tests

Alcohol may be detected in breath-collecting devices often carried by law enforcers.

Chapter 14: Point-of-Care Testing (Waived Tests)

While these simple tests have relatively lower risks of false results, it does not mean these are completely foolproof. To ensure the accuracy of test results, personnel must follow proper guidelines when performing these tests.

Since these tests are simple, CMS proficiency testing is not required at waived testing sites. However, there are certain circumstances when CMS includes inspection of waived testing procedures. These include the following situations:

- When a complaint has been raised
- To ascertain whether these sites are performing only the tests they are permitted to (i.e., certified waived tests)
- To gather data on waived tests

Test Preparations

Ensure the following:

- Workspaces are clean and safe.
- The test area is well lit.
- Patient privacy may be maintained.
- Storage requirements are being followed.
- Temperature logs are updated every day.
- Test kits and reagents are still within their validity dates; discard any past expiration dates.
- Contaminated, discolored or damaged test reagents are discarded.
- Test kit reagents are prepared following the manufacturer's instructions.
- Chilled reagents are allowed to be at room temperature before proceeding.
- All equipment is in working condition.
- All equipment is calibrated regularly following manufacturer instructions.

Manufacturer's Instructions

These are specific rules recommended by the manufacturer specific to a test kit. These vary among different manufacturers, even for the same tests. These may even vary for different lots or shipments of a test kit from the same manufacturer.

Always ensure that you are following the current instructions. Have a copy ready in the testing area for quick reference.

When receiving a new lot of test kits or a new shipment, always read the enclosed instructions for any changes. Inform your colleagues and supervisor if there are any.

Before proceeding with the test, ensure you have read and understood the instructions. If there are any clarifications, contact the manufacturer.

Follow the OSHA guidelines with every test procedure.

Off-Label Testing

Certain situations may allow modifications of test kits for purposes other than what is written in the manufacturer's instructions. This is referred to as "off-label." This means that the FDA did not clear the test kit for this off-label purpose, or the manufacturer did not have enough data to support this.

An example is testing capillary blood glucose using the glucometer when the patient's hematocrit level or oxygen saturation is not within the range described in the manufacturer's instructions. This is an off-label use and may result in unnecessary clinical interventions, which may harm the patient.

Quality Control

To ensure accurate test results, tests and equipment are regularly subjected to quality-control testing. Procedures are enclosed within the manufacturer's instructions.

When a quality-control test shows an incorrect result, you should:

- Troubleshoot the equipment.
- Check the expiration dates of reagents and test kits.
- Inspect reagents and test kits for contamination.
- Check compliance with storage requirements.
- Review the examiner's techniques for errors.

A control may be internal or external.

An **internal or procedural control** determines whether a test is working correctly, the sample size is adequate, and when applicable, the electronic functions of the equipment are in proper working condition.

An **external control** determines whether a test is performed properly and whether the results fall within the expected range. External controls are provided by the manufacturer (may be included or sold separately). These appear like test samples but may require processing before use.

Quality-control testing is scheduled regularly with consideration to the following:

- Manufacturer instructions
- When checking the validity of the test
- After environmental changes (such as electrical outages and refrigerator issues)
- For every trainee or new personnel who will be performing the test
- With every shipment of test kits or test reagents

Properly document the quality-control results. Documentation can help identify, track and address any problems with a test's integrity and performance.

When the quality-control results are incorrect, all patient test results should be withheld until the problem has been identified and addressed. Troubleshooting often involves:

- Rechecking compliance with manufacturer instructions
- Looking at the reagent and controls for contamination
- Rechecking compliance with storage requirements
- Checking the expiration date
- Following the manufacturer's troubleshooting instructions

If the problem still cannot be resolved by the above measures, contact the manufacturer or their assigned technicians.

Once the problem has been identified and addressed, repeat the quality-control testing. When the results are correct, repeat all patient samples and report their results.

The Test Procedure

Ensure that test requisitions are received, the patient is properly informed and has consented and the patient is identified with two verifiers.

Ensure that patients have complied with pretest requirements, such as fasting or abstaining from their medications.

Prepare your materials and ensure the test kits and reagents have not expired and have not been contaminated.

Read and understand the manufacturer's instructions; reference them quickly before proceeding with the test.

Collect and Handle the Samples Properly

Waived tests should be done only on unprocessed samples, such as:

- Whole blood (from dermal punctures or venipuncture)
- Anticoagulated blood
- Urine
- Feces
- Swabs either from the throat or nasopharynx
- Saliva
- Gastric tissue biopsy

Collection Devices

Ensure the use of the appropriate collection devices. When a collection device is included in the test kits, always use this. This ensures that the correct volumes are delivered, or the proper additives are present for the test.

Swabs may be included in the test kits. These are not interchangeable with other sterile swabs. The differences in the material may provide inaccurate results.

Dermal puncture and venipuncture collection devices are for single use only. A dermal puncture collection device comes in sizes corresponding to the patient population; choose the appropriate size for the patient.

Label Samples

Label each sample appropriately as soon as you collect it. Label the device before sample collection.

Run the Test

Since this is a waived test, you may be assigned to perform these tests after proper training. Running the test involves:

- Performing the tests exactly as indicated in the manufacturer's instructions.
- Quality-control testing.
- Using a timer, read results only after the indicated time interval has passed.

- Reading the results and recording these.
- Reporting the results.

Reading a result before the indicated time leads to an invalid or false negative test. There has not been enough time for the sample and reagent to complete their chemical reaction.

Reading a result after the indicated time leads to a false positive test, as colors may overdevelop or a false negative test, as colors fade. The reaction may also move beyond the visible window on the test cassette, leading to an invalid test. These depend on the test kit used.

When interpreting the results, utilize the color charts or reference guides provided by the manufacturer (when available).

Tests may be quantitative (provides a numeric value), qualitative (indicates only either positive or negative or invalid) or a mix of both.

When Results Are Invalid

Do not report the test results.

The tests should be repeated for instances when:

- A test indicates "invalid."
- It does not coincide with a patient's clinical presentation.
- Quantitative values are beyond the provided range.

Test equipment may also display a high or low result. Refer to the manufacturer's instructions for this situation. There should be additional steps to perform to arrive at accurate measurements. Once the problem has been identified and addressed, repeat all patient samples and report the corrected results.

Recording and Report Results

You are required to keep an organized log or record of all the test results for these waived tests. These should contain all the necessary information and be organized for ease of retrieval.

Guidelines for recording results are as follows:

- Quantitative values are recorded in standardized units.

- Qualitative results are recorded with words or letters rather than symbols (such as "Pos" to indicate positivity or "NR" to indicate "non-reactive").
- Invalid results are recorded as well, along with the results of the repeat test, but only report the correct result.

Guidelines for reporting results are as follows:

- They are in a standard format and reported promptly.
- Provide copies of test reports only to the patient or an authorized person.
- When reporting a result verbally (such as over the telephone), document this and promptly provide a written report.

Critical Values

Critical or panic values are results that need the physician's immediate attention.

Your laboratory or testing site must establish a clear system to communicate these critical values efficiently and promptly. These include:

- Defining the tests with panic values (such as glucose and potassium)
- Training staff on detecting critical values and alerting the physicians
- Having a communication system with the physician to promptly report panic values
- Documenting when and to whom a panic value has been reported

Confirmatory or Supplemental Testing

Waived test results may be equivocal. This may mean additional testing or a confirmatory test is required. Your laboratory may have its policies on when to perform confirmatory tests. This may need a referral to other laboratories that can perform higher complexity tests.

Refer to your policies for the necessary tests on how to order a confirmatory test, contact referral laboratories, collect samples and label and transport guidelines.

You are also required to document any referred testing. The records should contain the original test, the requested confirmatory test, the referral laboratory's name, the referral date and the date when the results are received.

Notifiable Diseases

Public health agencies have flagged certain diseases as "notifiable."

Testing sites are required to report confirmed positive or reactive results for infectious diseases, such as COVID-19, tuberculosis, active hepatitis, anthrax and botulism, among others.

Keep updated with your local public health agency for the current list of notifiable diseases.

Record-Keeping

Every laboratory should keep records of equipment logs, maintenance, quality-control documents and all test results for a certain period.

Keeping organized records facilitates retrieval and verification of information, assessment of test performance, troubleshooting and maintaining patient and personnel information. Record-keeping requirements vary with every state.

Chapter 15: Specimen Processing

Centrifugation and Aliquoting

Centrifugation

Laboratory tests may require either serum or plasma. A centrifuge is a machine that uses a high centrifugal force (at 850 to 1,000 gravity) to separate the blood cells from the serum or plasma component.

Whole blood from venipuncture may need to be spun for about 10 minutes inside a centrifuge.

Centrifugation must be completed within two hours of receiving the specimen to avoid analyte changes.

Serum is obtained after centrifugation of clotted blood. Blood collected in plain tubes or tubes containing serum separator gels or clot activators must be allowed to clot fully before centrifugation. A clot forms as quickly as five minutes (in a clot activator tube) or as late as one hour (from patients on anticoagulant medications).

Do not rim a clotted tube. This can lead to hemolysis.

Plasma is obtained after centrifugation of blood from anticoagulant-containing tubes.

Do not centrifuge a specimen for whole-blood analysis. Do not recentrifuge specimens. This can alter the test results.

Rules for Using a Centrifuge

Keep all tubes closed and balance the rotor by positioning tubes of equal size and volume across each other.

Always observe the centrifuge for any excessive vibration before leaving the area.

Keep the centrifuge covered when operating. This ensures that no aerosols or broken glass escape if a tube breaks inside the machine. If this happens, stop the centrifugation and unplug the appliance. Wear puncture-proof gloves when cleaning up the area of broken glass. Dispose of these in the sharps container. Disinfect the machine and tabletop with sodium hypochlorite.

Aliquoting

An aliquot refers to the part of a specimen transferred to another tube.

This procedure is done behind a plexiglass shield. Observe standard and airborne precautions. When opening a tube, cover the tops with gauze and uncap them with a twisting motion. Do not pop them off. Doing so can spray aerosols and leads to blood-borne pathogen exposure.

Always use a disposable pipette when aliquoting. Pouring the samples exposes you to aerosols.

Specimen Storage

Serum or plasma may be saved for a specified period under adequate conditions.

Room Temperature

Serum or plasma can be kept at room temperature (27° C) for up to 8 hours.

Refrigeration

Refrigerated serum or plasma should be maintained at 2° C to 8° C if testing is not done after eight hours. It can be kept for up to 48 hours.

Freezing

Freezing may be done if testing is expected to be done beyond 48 hours. This is achieved at temperatures of -20°C or lower. When a frozen sample has been thawed, it cannot be frozen again, as the cycle may destroy certain analytes.

Recommend Time for Specimen Testing

The CLSI has set the following limits to ensure accurate test results for the following tests:

APTT and Prothrombin Time

APTT specimens may remain at room temperature for up to four hours. Exception: for patients on heparin therapy, these tests should be separated within an hour and tested within four hours.

PT specimens may remain at room temperature for up to 24 hours. Chilling is not recommended, as it can activate factor VII.

Coagulation Tests

When a specimen for coagulation cannot be performed within four hours, plasma must be separated within an hour and frozen.

Complete Blood Count

A specimen in EDTA-anticoagulated tubes for **CBC** may remain at room temperature for up to 24 hours. Take note that for some tubes, a CBC should be done within six hours. However, from EDTA microtainers, a CBC should be done within four hours.

Erythrocyte Sedimentation Rate

Erythrocyte sedimentation rates should be analyzed after four hours of collection in EDTA tubes kept at room temperature. Refrigeration may extend this limit up to 12 hours.

Reticulocyte Count

Reticulocytes should be counted from six hours of collection in EDTA tubes kept at room temperature. Refrigeration may extend this limit up to 72 hours.

Glucose

A specimen in sodium fluoride tubes for **glucose** determinations may remain at room temperature for up to 24 hours. Refrigeration may extend this limit up to 48 hours.

Shipping Specimens

Transporting specimens over long distances from a nursing home or laboratory to another laboratory has been made possible by following certain regulations.

Categories of Infectious Substances

Biohazardous material may be designated as one of two classifications and regulated appropriately by the US Department of Transportation.

Category A. Exposure to these substances may be potentially disabling or life-threatening to humans (UN 2814) or animals. The classification is made based on the source's symptomatology and endemic conditions. For instance, *Bacillus anthracis* is classified as a Category A substance.

Category B. Exposure to these substances is not generally disabling or life-threatening to humans or animals. Most laboratory specimens fall in this category. For instance, newborn screening cards may be classified as a Category B substance (UN 3373).

Packaging and Labeling Requirements

The DOT strictly regulates the packaging and labeling of biohazardous material.

When shipped in public transport, they should be carried in **triple packaging**. The primary packaging should be leakproof and with a secure closure, such as tubes or screw-top cups. It should be enclosed in a second leak-proof container, such as a biohazard bag. The third should be a rigid container marked with "UN 3373 Biological Substance Category B."

The containers should be packed with Styrofoam and refrigerant packs to keep the samples cool.

Frozen samples should be packed in dry ice with an additional label indicating "Class 9 miscellaneous."

All specimens must be labeled completely and accompanied by their corresponding requisition forms.

Chapter 16: Laboratory Information Systems (LIS)

In the health care setting, computers are essential in managing large volumes of data for each patient.

Your duties involve utilizing electronic devices that:

- Facilitate identifying patients and printing labels at the bedside.
- Automatically transmit results to electronic records (portable point-of-care devices).
- Interface with the LIS and facilitate the transmission of data almost immediately after a machine has finished the test.
- Facilitate communication within the laboratory departments or throughout hospital wards and areas.

The LIS is a computer application developed explicitly for a laboratory's operation.

This application is capable of the following:

- Generating laboratory requisitions
- Preparing labels to be printed
- Monitoring the current status of a specimen, whether received, being processed or completed
- Interfacing with automated analyzers with which results are directly reported or verified
- Generating reports
- Storing an archive of a patient's health records
- Preparing bills for services
- Viewing results
- Monitoring compliance with quality-control procedures

Passwords

Password protection is an important way to regulate access to private patient records. You will be assigned your password. This authorizes you to create electronic transactions. Never share your password with anyone. All data within the LIS may be traced back to who has inputted it or handled the specimen.

Data Entry

Barcodes

This system of data entry automatically inputs information through a scanner. This method decreases the possibility of making clerical errors.

Radiofrequency ID

This system is similar to barcodes but uses a silicon chip instead of black-and-white lines. Its main advantage is its ability to detect from a distance of a hundred feet.

Current Procedure Terminology (CPT) Codes

These are codes necessary for laboratory tests to be reimbursed by insurance organizations. Certain facilities require you to input CPT codes corresponding to the tests requested into thc computer systems.

Chapter 17: Quality Management

Quality management refers to how a facility adheres to laboratory standards and evaluates the systems to prevent problems and resolve issues. It encompasses quality assessment and quality control.

Quality Assessment

This pertains to the laboratory's practices designed to guarantee quality patient care. It is overseen by The Joint Commission.

Documents of quality assessment include:

- Procedural manuals
  These provide a description of the principles and purpose for each test, specimen and collection requirements, a list of materials needed, special precautions (if any), procedure instructions, corrective actions, quality-control methods and reference ranges.

- Policies controlling and monitoring procedural variables
  Variable refers to any factor in the procedure that can be altered. This is classified according to when it may occur during the process: pre-examination, examination or post-examination.

- Reference manuals
  These are prepared for non-laboratory personnel or nurses assigned to certain specimen collections.

- Competency assessment
- Continuing education record

Record-keeping provides a means to evaluate the laboratory and make necessary changes to procedures, staff schedules and additional training.

Procedural Variables

Pre-examination variables include:

- Requisitioning errors, such as duplicate forms, missing forms
- Patient misidentification—the most critical error in the laboratory
- **Delta check**
  This compares a patient's old test results with the current results. A variation beyond the established parameter flags the result and alerts the personnel of a possible error.
- Equipment checks are necessary, as factory defects can result in unsatisfactory specimens.
- Patient preparation variables, as discussed in previous chapters
- Tourniquet application
- Site selection and preparation
- Venipuncture procedure
- Sharps and waste disposal
- Specimen transportation
- Specimen processing

Note: When a missed test has been discovered, this automatically becomes a STAT test.

Examination variables are important for phlebotomists when conducting a waived test or point-of-care test, as discussed in Chapter 14.

Post-examination variables include all activities directed toward reporting test results to the patient or physician. This may be accomplished by telephone, fax or electronic mail.

A laboratory report must include the following information:

- Patient identifiers (full names, birth date)
- Patient ID number
- Name of test performed
- Type of specimen
- Date and time of collection
- If a specimen was rejected, indicate its condition.
- Date and time of results
- Results of test
- Reference range or normal values

As the phlebotomist, you may be directly involved with reporting results. You may be assigned to deliver reports to the wards and place these inside a patient's chart. You may also be inputting written results into the laboratory information systems.

A misplaced or delayed report may potentially cause harm to the patient.

Electronically generated reports are more common. Nonetheless, ensure proper documentation of all results and keep permanent records available.

When reporting a result verbally (such as over the telephone), you must document the time and the name and designation of the caller. Promptly provide a written report.

Medical record-keeping is required for each patient. This includes all medications and procedures as well as laboratory results. Its purposes include:

- A reference for health care providers when formulating a patient care plan
- Documentation of all the communication that transpired among the health care staff
- Legal evidence
- Source of data for clinical research
- Documents to aid billing and quality-management systems reviews

Guidelines for documenting in a patient's chart:

- Use black ink.
- Sign your initials with the date and time of collection.
- Utilize only standardized abbreviations (when necessary).
- Write complete documentation of your actions as well as patient actions.
- To correct an error on paper, draw a single line across it and sign your initials.
- To correct an error online, do not erase the previous entry; instead, enter the updated result with a comment alerting users to the new entry.

Types of Quality Assessment

Quality assessment aids in reducing errors, improving patient safety and outcomes, ensuring employee safety and reducing overall costs. Either an internal or external assessment or a combination of both may be utilized for quality assessment.

An **internal assessment** involves processes for the staff to self-evaluate their current performance and practices. This method involves performing quality control, reviewing these along with the test results, evaluating record-keeping practices, documenting issues and creating an action plan to improve.

An **external assessment** involves a third party. They can perform the evaluation and offer training as well. This can be done by inviting colleagues or consultants who will evaluate current practices and record-keeping systems and point out areas for improvement.

This can also be done through proficiency testing programs.

A proficiency test is not required for CLIA-waived testing. This program regularly sends challenge samples to the enrolled laboratories to test as if they were patient samples. The program receives the results and compares these with their known values. The laboratory receives a report of how well they fared.

Quality-Management Systems

Quality assurance in phlebotomy is an integral component of laboratory quality management aligned with the requirements of The Joint Commission, CAP and CMS CLIA.

The first step in laboratory quality-management systems involves determining, evaluating and analyzing the workflow pathway. Every staff member involved in the laboratory workflow knows and understands their duties.

Turnaround Time

This refers to the length of time that transpires from the moment a test is requisitioned to the moment its results are generated and reported. This is determined by each facility. Monitoring the turnaround time for both STAT and routine requests allows laboratories to locate areas of concern and create an action plan to improve them.

Quality Systems Essentials, According to the CLSI

This forms the foundations of a quality-management system. This involves the interplay of the following 12 quality systems essentials (QSEs):

1. Assessment
2. Continuing improvement
3. Documents and records
4. Equipment
5. Facilities, safety
6. Information management
7. Nonconforming event management
8. Organization
9. Patient focus
10. Process management
11. Procurement and inventory
12. Staff

In compliance with quality-management systems, laboratories are required to develop a program to manage **nonconforming events**. This involves identifying issues within the laboratory workflow processes and improving them to provide better patient care and ensure the safety of patients and staff. It also includes the implementation of changes to these processes and procedures. Finally, it serves to investigate and remove the causes of these nonconforming events.

A **quality indicator** is presented through graphs that measure the performance of the laboratory processes. This aids in evaluating quality systems essentials in the laboratory.

Some examples of quality indicators in phlebotomy include:

- Lacking information on requisition forms
- Improper patient identification
- Improper timing of specimen collections
- Improper labeling of specimens
- Inappropriate handling of specimens
- Accidental needlesticks

The Lean System

This is designed to decrease costs and eliminate waste, allowing the laboratory to perform better with less and increasing customer and staff satisfaction. It involves six steps:

1. Sorting
2. Straightening
3. Scrubbing
4. Safety
5. Standardizing
6. Sustaining

The Six Sigma

This is adopted by The Joint Commission to guide laboratory facilities. Its main goal is to reduce errors to the acceptable level of 3.4 defects for every million opportunities. A laboratory that arrives at the Six Sigma level has addressed the most important variables for quality patient care.

This is achieved through the following methods:

- Defining objectives and current practices
- Measuring current practices and collecting data
- Analyzing the data to identify causation
- Improving current practices with this data
- Controlling the correction of issues within the data

Root Cause Analysis

This is a tool recommended for use by The Joint Commission when investigating sentinel events.

A sentinel event refers to an unexpected serious injury, often leading to death in the context of health care provision.

Sentinel Events

- Assaults, rape, homicides
- Fall
- Hemolytic transfusion reactions
- Medication errors
- Treatment delays
- Unexpected full-term neonatal death
- Retained foreign body following surgery

These events should be reported to The Joint Commission as soon as the event arises. They should also be documented for laboratory accreditation purposes. This report provides the following information:

- A description of the sentinel event
- A root cause analysis detailing the actions that could have caused the event
- A detailed action plan

The root cause analysis begins with investigating and reconstructing the event's details to outline the actions that could have caused it. The analysis is meant to focus on the failures of the workflow procedures and not on the staff's mistakes.

The Joint Commission analyzes each report it receives and sends alerts to other health care facilities regarding common areas from which issues arise.

A significant proportion of these events involve improper patient identification. This reiterates the importance of the first step in every phlebotomy procedure. Closely related to this is the proper labeling of samples, especially in blood banks.

Chapter 18: Cardiopulmonary Resuscitation

While your main responsibility is performing venipunctures and collecting specimens, there may be times when you are the first responder to a cardiac arrest. It is important to assess each patient.

Assessing Unconsciousness

As discussed in the earlier chapters, when you meet sleeping patients, you should wake them up politely. Unconscious or deceased patients may also appear to be peacefully asleep.

If it is difficult to rouse a patient, try making a loud noise, shaking them or pinching their earlobe. If the person does not respond, elicit pain by performing a sternal rub.

To perform this, make a fist and, using your knuckles, firmly rub the patient's mid-sternum up and down.

A semiconscious person may react by localizing to the pain or some subtle movement. In this situation, notify the nurse and physician for appropriate management.

If the patient is unresponsive, call for help immediately. Do not leave the patient. Perform the initial survey while waiting for help to arrive.

Initial Survey

Check the patient's airway by tilting the chin slightly upward and opening the mouth. If something is lodged, position the patient on their side and remove the obstruction. Otherwise, check for breathing by listening for breath sounds next to the patient's mouth and simultaneously watching their chest for movement.

If the patient is unresponsive and not breathing, immediately begin chest compressions.

Adult Cardiopulmonary Response

Chest Compressions

To perform chest compressions, place both hands interlaced on the patient's lower sternum. Using the heel of the hand, push on the sternum to depress it at least two inches. Allow the chest to recoil fully. This manually pumps the heart to allow blood to circulate. The rate should be in the range of 100 to 120 per minute.

In the hospital, there will be staff available to take over after this point. It is important to learn the steps, as you may be needed to assist throughout.

Rescue Breaths

While chest compressions are being given, generally for about two minutes per responder, another staff member attaches a bag-valve mask to the patient to provide rescue breaths. It should be given at a rate of one per six seconds.

Cardiopulmonary Resuscitation Modifications

Infant (Under 12 Months Old)

To perform chest compressions on infants, place two fingers on the infant's sternum, just below the level of the nipples. The depth of compression is reduced to 1.5 inches. The rate of compressions remains at a range of 100 to 120 per minute.

If you are the lone responder, interrupt every cycle of 30 compressions to give two rescue breaths (using a valve device) until another staff member arrives.

Children (1 to 14 Years Old)

To perform chest compressions on children, place the heel of either one or two hands (considering the child's size) on the child's lower sternum. Similar to adult compressions, the compression depth is two inches and the rate of compressions remains at a range of 100 to 120 per minute.

If you are the lone responder, interrupt every cycle of 30 compressions to give two rescue breaths (using a valve device) until the other staff arrive.

Appendix: Table of Laboratory Tests

Blood Culture Bottles or Yellow SPS Tubes

DIAGNOSTIC TEST	REMARKS	DEPARTMENT	CLINICAL CORRELATION
Blood cultures	Keep at room temperature; aseptic technique.	Microbiology	Sepsis

Gray Tubes

DIAGNOSTIC TEST	REMARKS	DEPARTMENT	CLINICAL CORRELATION
Ethanol/alcohol	Keep the tube closed; it may be subjected to a chain of custody; remember to use a nonalcohol-based skin cleanser in preparing the site.	Chemistry	Intoxication
Lactate	Test immediately (within 15 minutes); avoid hemolysis; do not use a tourniquet.	Chemistry	Muscular disorders
Fasting blood sugar (FBS)	Confirm that the patient adequately fasted for 8 hours.	Chemistry	Diabetes; monitoring blood sugar control
Glucose		Chemistry	Hypoglycemia or hyperglycemia

Pink Tubes

DIAGNOSTIC TEST	REMARKS	DEPARTMENT	CLINICAL CORRELATION
Antibody screen	BB identification	Blood bank	Blood transfusion
ABO and Rh Blood typing	BB identification	Blood bank	Identify blood type

Crossmatch	BB identification remains on 72 hours	Blood bank	Blood compatibility
Type and screen	BB identification	Blood bank	Blood transfusion

Lavender Tubes

DIAGNOSTIC TEST	REMARKS	DEPARTMENT	CLINICAL CORRELATION
Adrenocorticotropic hormone (ACTH)	Freeze plasma.	Chemistry	Adrenal and pituitary gland function
Ammonia	Do not use gel tubes.	Chemistry	Hepatic encephalopathy
Antidiuretic hormone	Freeze plasma.	Chemistry	Pituitary function
Brain natriuretic peptide (BNP)	Remains stable for only 4 hours.	Chemistry	Congestive heart failure
Carbon monoxide	Do not underfill; needs immediate refrigeration.	Chemistry	Carbon monoxide toxicity
Cryoglobulin	Use warmed tubes and transport at 37° C.	Chemistry	Vasculitides, glomerulonephritis, macroglobulinemias
Homocysteine (Hcy)	Send in an ice slurry.	Chemistry	Methionine metabolism disorder
Hemoglobin electrophoresis		Chemistry	Hgb abnormalities
Hemoglobin A1c		Chemistry	Diabetes mellitus
Parathyroid hormones (PTH)	Send in an ice slurry.	Chemistry	Hypercalcemia, Hypoparathyroidism, Hyperparathyroidism
Myocardial infarction panel (includes creatine kinase MB, myoglobins and troponins)	Remains stable for only 4 hours.	Chemistry	MI
Complete blood count		Hematology	Infection, hematopoietic disorders, leukemias, anemia
White blood cell (WBC) count		Hematology	Infections or leukemias

Differential (Diff)	Create peripheral blood smear within an hour of collecting.	Hematology	Infections, anemia, leukemias, blood dyscrasias
Hematocrit (Hgb)		Hematology	Anemias
Hemoglobin (Hct)		Hematology	Anemias
Red blood cell (RBC) count		Hematology	Anemias
Reticulocyte count (Retic)		Hematology	Anemias; bone marrow function
Sickle cell screen		Hematology	Sickle cell crises
Erythrocyte sedimentation rate	The tube must be at least half full.	Hematology	Inflammatory disorders
Glucose-6-phosphate dehydrogenase		Hematology	G6PD-deficiency
Platelet aggregation		Hematology	Test of platelet function
Coombs test (direct)		Blood bank	Anemias or Rh incompatibility
T-cell count		Immuno-serology	Immune function/HIV monitoring
Viral load	Keep plasma frozen.	Immuno-serology	HIV monitoring

Light-Blue with Thrombin

DIAGNOSTIC TEST	REMARKS	DEPARTMENT	CLINICAL CORRELATION
Fibrin degradation product (FDP)	Fill only up to the 2 mL mark; it must clot immediately.	Coagulation	Disseminated intravascular coagulation

Light-Blue Tubes

DIAGNOSTIC TEST	REMARKS	DEPARTMENT	CLINICAL CORRELATION
Antithrombin III	Keep plasma frozen.	Coagulation	Clotting disorders
DIC panel		Coagulation	Coagulation systems
D-Dimer (D-DI)	Full tube (remains stable for only 4 hours)	Coagulation	DIC; thrombotic disorders
Heparin anti-Xa		Coagulation	Therapeutic monitoring for heparin
International normalized ratios	Full tubes	Coagulation	Therapeutic monitoring for Coumadin
Activated partial thromboplastin time	Tubes must be full; centrifuge heparinized specimen within 1 hour; stable for 4 hours at room temperature.	Coagulation	Therapeutic monitoring for heparin; clotting disorders
Plasminogen		Coagulation	Clotting disorders
Prothrombin time	Tubes must be full; stable for 24 hrs at room temperature.	Coagulation	Therapeutic monitoring for Coumadin; clotting disorders
Platelet aggregation		Hematology	Test of platelet function
Factor assays	Full tubes	Chemistry	Detect specific clotting factor function
Fibrinogen	Full tubes	Chemistry	Coagulation disorders

Royal Blue (Serum or Plain)

DIAGNOSTIC TEST	REMARKS	DEPARTMENT	CLINICAL CORRELATION
Aluminum (Al)	Serum (plain)	Chemistry	Aluminum toxicity
Zinc	Serum (plain)	Chemistry	Zinc deficiency
Chromium (Cr)	Separate and needs immediate refrigeration	Chemistry	To monitor prosthetic implants
Copper		Chemistry	Biliary cirrhosis

Royal Blue (EDTA)

DIAGNOSTIC TEST	REMARKS	DEPARTMENT	CLINICAL CORRELATION
Chromium (Cr)	Separate and needs immediate refrigeration	Chemistry	To monitor prosthetic implants
Lead (Pb)	Collect in EDTA.	Chemistry	Neurological function

Tan Tubes

DIAGNOSTIC TEST	REMARKS	DEPARTMENT	CLINICAL CORRELATION
Lead (Pb)	Collect in EDTA.	Chemistry	Neurological function

Light Green (Plasma Separator Tube)

DIAGNOSTIC TEST	REMARKS	DEPARTMENT	CLINICAL CORRELATION
Porphyrins	Photosensitive; wrap tubes in aluminum foil to shield them from light.	Chemistry	Porphyria cutanea tarda
Myocardial infarction panel (includes creatine kinase	Remains stable for only 4 hours.	Chemistry	MI

MB, myoglobins and troponins)			

Green (Non-Gel)

DIAGNOSTIC TEST	REMARKS	DEPARTMENT	CLINICAL CORRELATION
Vitamin B6	Do not collect in gel barrier tubes; confirm that the patient adequately fasted; photosensitive; wrap tubes in aluminum foil to shield from light.	Chemistry	Hypophosphatasia
pH	Send in an ice slurry.	Chemistry	Acid-base balance

White (Plasma Preparation Tube)

DIAGNOSTIC TEST	REMARKS	DEPARTMENT	CLINICAL CORRELATION
Myocardial infarction panel (includes creatine kinase MB, myoglobins and troponins)	Remains stable for only 4 hours.	Chemistry	MI
Viral load	Keep plasma frozen.	Immunoserology	HIV monitoring
Brain natriuretic peptide (BNP)	Remains stable for only 4 hours.	Chemistry	Congestive heart failure

Either SST Tubes (Red or Gold Gel Tubes) or Plasma Separator Tubes (Light Green)

DIAGNOSTIC TEST	REMARKS	DEPARTMENT	CLINICAL CORRELATION
Potassium		Chemistry	Muscular function, cardiac function
Aspartate aminotransferase		Chemistry	Hepatic disease, cardiac muscle damage
Alanine aminotransferase		Chemistry	Hepatic disease
Alkaline phosphatase		Chemistry	Bone disorders
Amylase	Transport in an ice slurry.	Chemistry	Pancreatitis
Albumin		Chemistry	Malnutrition; hepatic disease
Beta human chorionic gonadotropin		Chemistry	Pregnancy, testicular cancer
Blood urea nitrogen (BUN)		Chemistry	Renal disorders
Calcium	Immediate refrigeration	Chemistry	Skeletal disorders
Cholesterol		Chemistry	Coronary artery disease
Creatine kinase (CK)		Chemistry	Myocardial infarction, muscular damage
Creatinine		Chemistry	Renal disorders
Electrolyte panel (sodium, potassium, chloride)	Keep at room temperature.	Chemistry	Fluid and acid-base balance
Ferritin		Chemistry	Iron deficiency
Iron		Chemistry	Anemia
Lactate dehydrogenase		Chemistry	MI
Lipoprotein cholesterols (HDL, LDL, VLDL)		Chemistry	Dyslipidemia, cardiovascular disease
Phosphorus		Chemistry	Endocrine and bone disorders

Thyroid-stimulating hormone, FT4, FT3		Chemistry	Thyroid function
Triglycerides		Chemistry	Coronary heart disease
Iron-binding capacity		Chemistry	Anemia
Bilirubin, total and direct (Bili)	Photosensitive	Chemistry	Hepatic, hemolytic disorders
Digoxin		Chemistry	Heart stimulant
Lipase		Chemistry	Pancreatitis
Fasting blood sugar (FBS)	Fast for 8 hours.	Chemistry	Diabetes; blood sugar control
Glucose		Chemistry	Hypoglycemia or hyperglycemia
Sodium		Chemistry	Acid-base balance
Vitamin B12	Photosensitive	Chemistry	Anemia
Complement C3, C4 titers; haptoglobins		Immunoserology	Immune disorders, hemolytic anemias
Immunoglobulin titers (IgG, IgA, IgM)		Immunoserology	Immune system function

Plain Red Tubes

DIAGNOSTIC TEST	REMARKS	DEPARTMENT	CLINICAL CORRELATION
Antibiotic assays	Do not collect in gel barrier tubes.	Chemistry	Broad-spectrum antibiotics
Anti-HIV		Immunoserology	HIV
Antistreptolysin O (ASO) titer	Immediate refrigeration	Immunoserology	Rheumatic fever
Complement haptoglobins		Immunoserology	Immune disorders, hemolytic anemias
Immunoglobulin titers		Immunoserology	Immune system function
Calcitonin	Do not use gel; freeze serum immediately.	Chemistry	Medullary thyroid cancer
Carbamazepine (Tegretol)	Do not collect in gel barrier tubes.	Chemistry	Altered protein-binding capacity
Cold agglutinins	Maintain at 37° C; do not use gel.	Immunoserology	Atypical pneumonia
Cryoglobulin	Warmed tubes; transport at 37° C	Chemistry	Vasculitides, glomerulonephritis, macroglobulinemias
Drug screen	Do not use gel.	Chemistry	Detects recent drug use; identifies drug
Digoxin		Chemistry	Heart stimulant
Fasting blood sugar (FBS)	Fast for 8 hours.	Chemistry	Diabetes; blood sugar control
Glucose		Chemistry	Hypoglycemia or hyperglycemia
Febrile antibody panel		Immunoserology	Antibody screen for salmonella, brucella francisella, rickettsia
Salicylate (aspirin)	Do not collect in gel barrier tubes.	Chemistry	Salicylate toxicity
Valproic acid (Depakote)	Do not collect in gel barrier tubes.	Chemistry	Valproic toxicity
Vitamin A	Do not collect in gel barrier tubes; it requires fasting.	Chemistry	Vitamin A deficiency and toxicity

Vitamin B12	Photosensitive	Chemistry	Anemia
Western blot		Immunoserology	HIV
Antiepileptic drugs	Do not use gel; centrifugation and separation within 1 hour.	Chemistry	Therapeutic monitoring

SST Tubes (Red or Gold Gel Tubes)

DIAGNOSTIC TEST	**REMARKS**	**DEPARTMENT**	**CLINICAL CORRELATION**
Acid phosphatase	Freeze serum.	Chemistry	Prostate cancer
Alpha-fetoprotein (AFP)		Chemistry	Testicular and ovarian cancers
Apolipoproteins (-A and -B)		Chemistry	Cardiac diseases
Brain natriuretic peptide (BNP)	Remains stable for only 4 hours.	Chemistry	Congestive heart failure
Carcinoembryonic antigen (CEA)		Chemistry	Malignancy
Complement levels		Chemistry	Immune system function/ autoimmune disorders
Creatine kinases (isoenzyme -MB, -MM, -BB)		Chemistry	Myocardial infarction, muscular damage, CNS damage
Gastrin	Send in an ice slurry.	Chemistry	Gastric cancer or pernicious anemias
Insulin		Chemistry	Function of pancreas
Prostate-specific Ag		Chemistry	Prostate cancer
Prostate acid phosphatase		Chemistry	Prostate cancer
Protein		Chemistry	Hepatic, renal, bone marrow, metabolic or

			nutritional disorder
Testosterone		Chemistry	Testicular function
Total protein (TP)		Chemistry	Renal and hepatic disorders
Troponins I and T		Chemistry	Myocardial function
Uric acid		Chemistry	Renal disorders, gout
Vitamin D		Chemistry	Calcium absorption
Viral load	Keep plasma frozen.	Immunoserology	HIV monitoring

Either SST Tubes (Red or Gold Gel Tubes) or Plain Red Tubes

DIAGNOSTIC TEST	REMARKS	DEPARTMENT	CLINICAL CORRELATION
Angiotensin-converting enzyme	Send in an ice slurry.	Chemistry	Sarcoidosis
C-peptide	Requires fasting; avoid hemolysis.	Chemistry	Hypoglycemia
CA-125	Keep refrigerated.	Chemistry	Ovarian cancer
Carotene, beta	Photosensitive;	Chemistry	Fat malabsorption
Cortisol	Serum only; timed (morning)	Chemistry	Adrenal cortex function
C-reactive protein		Chemistry	Inflammatory processes
Folate		Chemistry	Anemia
Gamma-glutamyl transpeptidase (GGT)		Chemistry	Hepatic disease
Ionized calcium (iCA2+)	Full tube	Chemistry	To confirm abnormal levels
Lithium (Li)	Draw 12 hours after giving the drug.	Chemistry	Therapeutic monitoring
Magnesium		Chemistry	Musculoskeletal disorders

Myoglobin		Chemistry	Muscle damage
Osmolality		Chemistry	Comatose patients
Protein electrophoresis		Chemistry	Multiple myeloma/ abnormal proteins
Anti-hepatitis A		Immunoserology	Hep A infection
Hepatitis B surface Ag		Immunoscrology	Hep B infection
Hep B core Ab		Immunoserology	Recent or previous Hep B infection
Hep B surface Ab		Immunoserology	Immunity to hepatitis B
Anti-hepatitis C		Immunoserology	Hep C infection
Antinuclear antibody (ANA)		Immunoserology	SLE; autoimmune disease
Epstein-Barr virus assay		Immunoserology	Infectious mononucleosis
Mononucleosis screen (Mono test)		Immunoserology	Infectious mononucleosis
Fluorescent treponemal antibody absorption		Immunoserology	Syphilis
Rapid plasmin reagin		Immunoserology	Syphilis
Venereal disease research laboratory		Immunoserology	Syphilis
Rubella immunoglobulin titers		Immunoserology	Immunity to rubella

Test 1 Questions

1) As today's health care system is evolving, some phlebotomists may be trained to perform additional duties, such as which of the following?

(A) Specimen transport.

(B) Dermal puncture.

(C) Taking vital signs.

(D) Selecting specimen containers.

2) Communicating effectively involves which of the following?

(A) Tone of voice.

(B) Listening skills.

(C) Gestures.

(D) All of the above.

3) Consent is implied for an adult patient for blood extraction under which of the following conditions?

(A) They sign the consent form.

(B) They extend their left arm.

(C) They nod in agreement.

(D) There is a witness present.

4) Being sensitive to cultural diversity is a desirable professional trait in the health care staff. A phlebotomist can respond appropriately by doing which of the following?

(A) Stereotyping patients.

(B) Noticing the patient's reactions and accommodating them.

(C) Examining the patient's arm very quickly.

(D) Invading the patient's personal space.

5) Which of the following is a federal law that stipulates the confidentiality of patient information?

(A) CLIA.

(B) CLSI.

(C) TJC.

(D) HIPAA.

6) Agents of infections are described as linked together to form a chain. A susceptible host may, in turn, become which of the following?

(A) Portal of exit.

(B) Mode of transmission.

(C) Reservoir.

(D) Infectious agent.

7) You are assigned to collect dermal punctures for newborn spot tests. Before you enter the neonatal ICU, which of the following is your priority?

(A) Greeting the nurses.

(B) Washing your hands.

(C) Donning a gown and gloves.

(D) Putting on a mask.

8) Which of the following is the proper sequence for removing PPE?

(A) The most contaminated items are removed first.

(B) The least contaminated items are removed first.

(C) The first PPE worn is removed first.

(D) The last PPE worn is removed first.

9) Before meeting any patient, which of the following is the routine policy OSHA encourages for controlling the spread of infection?

(A) Emergency precautions.

(B) Standard precautions.

(C) Universal precautions.

(D) Blood-borne precautions.

10) Which of the following types of waste refers to objects that may cut or puncture?

(A) Pathologic/anatomical.

(B) Recyclable.

(C) Chemical.

(D) Sharp.

11) To correctly don PPEs, all except which of the following equipment must be available?

(A) Waste bin.

(B) Mask.

(C) Face shield.

(D) Size-appropriate gloves.

12) Which of the following is a specialized tissue that provides a scaffold for the organs?

(A) Epithelial.

(B) Connective.

(C) Muscular.

(D) Nervous.

13) The elbow lies proximal to the hand. This means that the elbow is which of the following?

(A) Nearer to the center of the body than the hand.

(B) Farther to the center of the body than the hand.

(C) Toward the midline of the hand.

(D) On the side of the hand.

14) Which of the following planes cuts the body into an anterior and posterior section?

(A) Frontal.

(B) Sagittal.

(C) Midsagittal.

(D) Transverse.

15) The ventral cavities contain all except which of the following organs and subcavities?

(A) Thoracic.

(B) Abdominal.

(C) Cranial.

(D) Pelvic.

16) Which of the following is a large artery branching near the aorta and is often used as a site for identifying pulse in the event of an emergency?

(A) Radial.

(B) Carotid.

(C) Superior vena cava.

(D) Pulmonary.

17) Which of the following occurs when the body uses up a lot of clotting factors as a result of coagulation happening everywhere in the body due to several infected injuries?

(A) Disseminated intravascular coagulation.

(B) Hemophilia.

(C) Deep vein thrombosis.

(D) Clot lysis.

18) Where is the pulse commonly felt?

(A) The neck, elbow crease, and wrists.

(B) The chest, neck, and thigh.

(C) The forearm, hands, and knee.

(D) The neck, below the thumb, and the sides of the forehead.

19) Which of the following are considered the most common leukocyte found in the body?

(A) Lymphocytes.

(B) Neutrophils.

(C) Monocytes.

(D) Basophils.

20) Which of the following is a term attributed to the pain and swelling of a vein that develops as a result of carelessness when doing phlebotomy work?

(A) Phlebitis.

(B) Thrombosis.

(C) Aneurysm.

(D) Arteriosclerosis.

21) Which of the following tests is used to evaluate the function of the extrinsic coagulation pathway?

(A) Activated partial thromboplastin time.

(B) Prothrombin time.

(C) Thrombin Time.

(D) D-dimer.

22) Blood pressure determines the pressure subjected to the blood vessel walls during the systole and diastole. It is reported as two readings in millimeters of mercury. Which of the following is the number written above?

(A) Systolic blood pressure.

(B) Diastolic blood pressure.

(C) Pulse rate.

(D) Pulse pressure.

23) Which of the following blood vessels carries deoxygenated blood?

(A) Pulmonary vein.

(B) Carotid artery.

(C) Pulmonary artery.

(D) Aorta.

24) The contents of a phlebotomy tray include all except which of the following?

(A) ETS.

(B) Tourniquet.

(C) Urine cups.

(D) Syringe.

25) EDTA prevents blood from clotting through which of the following actions?

(A) Releasing heparin.

(B) Binding calcium.

(C) Binding thrombin.

(D) Binding fibrinogen.

26) Which of the following evacuated tubes is coated with an additive that inhibits thrombin?

(A) Lavender.

(B) Green.

(C) Black.

(D) Yellow.

27) Which of the following chemicals is added to tubes to prevent glycolysis?

(A) Na heparin.

(B) Na fluoride.

(C) Na polyanethol sulfate.

(D) Na citrate.

28) A requisition form is valid if received through which of the following?

(A) The patient.

(B) The pneumatic tube system.

(C) The hospital information system.

(D) All of the above.

29) Before proceeding with a venipuncture, you must do which of the following?

(A) Read out the patient's name; check if they nod or say yes.

(B) Ask every patient to verbally state their first and last names and birth date.

(C) Check only the patient's ID band with the requisition form.

(D) Check only the ID numbers, since this is reliable.

30) You find out that a patient has not complied with fasting requirements for a blood cholesterol determination. You inform the nurse. She says to go ahead with the procedure. You should do which of the following?

(A) Argue with the nurse.

(B) Report the nurse to your supervisor.

(C) Draw the blood as instructed and make sure to note "not fasting" on the requisition form.

(D) Wait to hear the instructions directly from the physician.

31) The butterfly system preferred for use in venipuncture on which of the following patients?

(A) A 70-year-old active man.

(B) A 24-year-old undergoing chemotherapy.

(C) A 30-year-old businesswoman.

(D) A 15-year-old boy.

32) When necessary, small veins on the dorsum of the hand can be used for venipuncture. Which of the following blood collection systems is best for this area?

(A) Winged collection system.

(B) Syringe system.

(C) ETS.

(D) Never be used.

33) A tourniquet was used to find the vein. How long is the interval before it can be reapplied to draw the blood?

(A) 60 seconds.

(B) 120 seconds.

(C) 180 seconds.

(D) 5 minutes.

34) Where is the proper position of the tourniquet on the patient's arm?

(A) At least 2 inches above the elbow crease.

(B) At least 1 or 2 inches superior to the antecubital fossa.

(C) At least 3 or 4 inches superior to the antecubital fossa.

(D) Applied securely around a joint or bony area.

35) What happens when the patient is allowed to pump their fist while you are extracting blood?

(A) Hemolysis.

(B) Hemoconcentration.

(C) Hematoma.

(D) Skin blanching.

36) As blood flows down the tube, the phlebotomist should do which of the following?

(A) Instruct the patient to pump their fist.

(B) Instruct the patient to open their fist.

(C) Tighten the tourniquet.

(D) Loosen the tourniquet.

37) When the patient's elbow is allowed to bend over the site without applying adequate pressure, which of the following happens?

(A) Hemolysis.

(B) Hemoconcentration.

(C) Hematoma.

(D) Skin blanching.

38) Which of the following are important data to write on the specimen labels?

(A) Patient ID number.

(B) The requesting physician's name and signature.

(C) Test(s) requested.

(D) Special handling requirements for the tests requested.

39) Which of the following statements on the consequences of improper transport is true?

(A) Glycolysis causes falsely high blood glucose values.

(B) Hemolysis causes falsely low serum potassium values.

(C) Coagulation factors are increased at room temperature.

(D) Bilirubin is photosensitive; the tube must be wrapped in foil during transport.

40) You are asked to do a venipuncture on a comatose patient. There is no ID band on the patient. Which of the following actions is appropriate?

(A) Ask the other patients in the ward to identify the patient.

(B) Postpone the procedure; leave the requisition with the nurses.

(C) Wait for a family member.

(D) Find the nurse to attach an ID band to the patient.

41) It is acceptable to have another person verify a patient's identity when the patient is which of the following?

(A) A teenager.

(B) Elderly.

(C) Cognitively impaired.

(D) Combative.

42) Why are most routine venipunctures often collected early in the morning?

(A) The physicians make rounds in the morning and need these results early.

(B) The patient is well-rested and fasting.

(C) The patient will have already had breakfast.

(D) Fewer adverse reactions (i.e., nausea, fainting) are encountered.

43) Preexamination variables are those that affect the integrity of the specimens and alter test results. Which of the following statements is correct?

(A) When a patient has not complied with fasting, you must cancel the venipuncture.

(B) Patients should lie down for 30 minutes before drawing blood for aldosterone tests.

(C) Following short-term exercise, test results are unaffected.

(D) At higher altitudes, oxygen and hemoglobin levels are lower.

44) Your patient suddenly starts to have a seizure while you are collecting blood. Which of the following should you do first?

(A) Remove the tourniquet and needle, apply pressure to the site, and summon help.

(B) Forcibly restrain the patient.

(C) Run to the nurse station to summon help.

(D) Turn the patient's head to one side and insert a tongue depressor in the mouth.

45) Hemoconcentration is produced by which of the following?

(A) Performing venipuncture on sclerotic veins.

(B) Removing the tourniquet before 1 minute.

(C) Failing to instruct the patient to pump their fist.

(D) Inverting the evacuated tubes.

46) Which of the following areas are suitable for venipuncture?

(A) Below a hematoma.

(B) Above a hematoma.

(C) Sclerosed veins.

(D) Healed burns or scars.

47) When attempting venipuncture on a dialysis patient with an AV graft, you should do which of the following?

(A) Apply the tourniquet 3 inches below the AV graft.

(B) Collect blood from the AV graft.

(C) Collect blood from the other arm.

(D) Only A and B.

48) Which of the following needle positions causes hematoma by puncturing the veins through the tissue?

(A) Bevel too close to the vessel wall.

(B) Needle advanced too deep into the vein.

(C) Needle angle too narrow.

(D) Needle not inside the vein.

49) Which of the following technical errors leads to a hematoma formation?

(A) Releasing the tourniquet before withdrawing the needle.

(B) Applying pressure to the site.

(C) Using a large needle on a small vein.

(D) All of the above.

50) Which of the following can cause a specimen to be rejected?

(A) Clotted red tubes.

(B) Using a partial-draw tube.

(C) Incompletely filling an SST.

(D) Clotted lavender tubes.

51) On which patient population is a dermal puncture appropriate?

(A) Cancer patients on chemotherapy.

(B) Elderly patients.

(C) Patients on glucose monitoring.

(D) All of the above.

52) Which of the following tests may be run on capillary blood?

(A) ESR.

(B) Blood culture.

(C) Coagulation tests.

(D) Newborn screening test.

53) Capillary blood contains higher levels of which of the following analytes?

(A) Potassium.

(B) Albumin.

(C) Glucose.

(D) Calcium.

54) An improper dermal puncture, which fails to cut perpendicular to the fingerprint, will do which of the following?

(A) Cause significant discomfort to the patient.

(B) Cause blood to collect and flow in the grooves.

(C) Contaminate the sample.

(D) Hemolyze the sample.

55) Which of the following is a correct practice when performing dermal punctures?

(A) Restrain every pediatric patient, as they might be uncooperative.

(B) Promise that the procedure will be quick and painless.

(C) Make a note of agitation and crying in the requisition form.

(D) It is unnecessary to document consent when a child is simply wrapped in a blanket for the dermal puncture.

56) Why is warming the site recommended in dermal puncture?

(A) It prevents hemolysis.

(B) It increases blood flow.

(C) It prevents the formation of microclots.

(D) It is soothing for the patient.

57) Why do most tests require wiping off the first drop of blood when collecting dermal puncture specimens?

(A) It avoids contamination.

(B) It increases blood flow.

(C) It prevents the formation of a round drop of blood.

(D) It prevents blood-borne infections.

58) Which of the following is a condition caused by the lack of an enzyme to break down a sugar found in milk and results in an accumulation in the blood?

(A) Phenylketonuria.

(B) Galactosemia.

(C) Cystic fibrosis.

(D) Congenital hypothyroidism.

59) Which of the following statements describes a properly collected newborn screen sample?

(A) Using one drop of blood from a heel puncture to fill and soak one circle.

(B) Using multiple drops of blood to fill and soak one circle.

(C) Using a capillary pipette to apply a uniform drop of blood on each circle.

(D) Applying one drop of blood to each side of the filter paper.

60) On which area should you view the slide under the microscope to ensure that your sample is representative of the patient's blood?

(A) On the feathered edge.

(B) Around the holes.

(C) At the thickest area.

(D) At the creases.

61) Which of the following refers to the bacteria in the bloodstream causing symptoms of fever and tachycardia?

(A) Sepsis.

(B) Bacteremia.

(C) Meningitis.

(D) Allergy.

62) Which of the following is the ideal time for collecting a blood culture?

(A) After the height of fever.

(B) Just before the height of fever.

(C) After giving antibiotics.

(D) During a patient's basal state.

63) When it is necessary to take a blood culture sample from patients who are already taking antibiotics, you must do which of the following?

(A) Ask the nurse to discontinue the patient's antibiotics for 24 hours.

(B) Collect the sample in special bottles containing activated charcoal.

(C) Ensure that the patient has taken activated charcoal first.

(D) Ask the nurse to skip the patient's antibiotics right before your collection.

64) Which of the following is a suitable cleanser for clearing bacteria off the skin in a newborn?

(A) Chlorhexidine gluconate.

(B) 70% isopropyl alcohol.

(C) 40% isopropyl alcohol.

(D) ChloraPrep swabs.

65) Which of the following is the correct blood culture volume requirement for infants weighing less than 5 kilograms?

(A) 1 to 3 mL of blood per pediatric bottle.

(B) 0.5 mL of blood per pediatric bottle.

(C) 1 mL in only one pediatric bottle.

(D) only 0.5 mL per kilogram.

66) A chilled specimen should not be used for which of the following tests?

(A) Arterial blood gases.

(B) Serum potassium.

(C) ACTH.

(D) PTH.

67) Which of the following is true when collecting forensic samples for use in legal proceedings?

(A) The specimen must be collected in front of two witnesses.

(B) Only the physician may draw the blood.

(C) You should document your name and the date and time on the chain-of-custody form.

(D) You will be asked to identify the patient in court.

68) Which of the following may cause a falsely low blood alcohol level?

(A) Using 70% isopropyl alcohol as a skin cleanser.

(B) Underfilling the gray tube.

(C) Overfilling the gray tube.

(D) Using Zephiran chloride as a skin cleanser.

69) Which of the following characteristics would make a volunteer eligible to donate blood?

(A) 16 years old.

(B) weight of 48 kg.

(C) Blood pressure of 180/110 mmHg.

(D) Hemoglobin count of 13 g/dL.

70) Donor units are routinely tested for the presence of which of the following blood-borne pathogens?

(A) Human immunodeficiency virus.

(B) *Treponema pallidum.*

(C) HTLV.

(D) All of the above.

71) The gauge of the needle to collect blood should be which of the following?

(A) 16- or 17-gauge.

(B) 17- or 18-gauge.

(C) 23-gauge.

(D) 25-gauge.

72) Which of the following procedures allows a person to preemptively donate a unit of their blood to be transfused during or after the operation?

(A) Autologous donation.

(B) Heterologous donation.

(C) Homologous donation.

(D) Self-donation.

73) Following successful blood donation, volunteers should be instructed to do all except which of the following?

(A) Drink plenty of fluids.

(B) Avoid strenuous activities.

(C) Lie down if they feel dizzy or nauseous.

(D) Return to work involving lifting heavy objects.

74) Which of the following is a method of obtaining a sterile urine sample for bacterial cultures from patients who are bedridden or unable to void?

(A) Catheter collection.

(B) Use of a collection bag.

(C) Midstream clean-catch sample.

(D) First-morning void.

75) The correct method of collecting a nasopharyngeal swab involves which of the following?

(A) Immersing the swab in saline and mixing it vigorously.

(B) Crushing the contents of the ampule of transport media.

(C) Disposing of the swab, along with excess liquid.

(D) Transporting the swab to the laboratory on an ice slurry.

76) When using a pneumatic tube system, all except which of the following is correct?

(A) Tubes must be properly cushioned.

(B) Keep specimens in leak-proof biohazard containers.

(C) Tubes may be used to transport specimens collected through invasive means.

(D) All of the above.

77) Which of the following specimens may be used to investigate the organisms or crystals in the joints?

(A) Amniotic fluid.

(B) Synovial fluid.

(C) Cerebrospinal fluid.

(D) Serous fluid.

78) Which of the following CSF tube is correctly paired with its intended department?

(A) Tube 1 for chemistry.

(B) Tube 2 for microbiology.

(C) Tube 3 for hematology.

(D) All of the above.

79) Which of the following types of serous fluid is located between the membranes of the abdominal cavity?

(A) Pleural.

(B) Pericardial.

(C) Parietal.

(D) Peritoneal.

80) Malabsorption of lactose can be detected in the breath through which of the following tests?

(A) C-urea breath test.

(B) Hydrogen breath test.

(C) Alcohol breath test.

(D) Carbon dioxide breath test.

81) Which of the following is the correct instruction for patients before collecting sputum specimens?

(A) Do not eat or drink.

(B) Smoking is allowed.

(C) Swallow a glass of water right before expectorating.

(D) Take a sample right before going to bed.

82) The ideal time to centrifuge a specimen is which of the following?

(A) 2 hours after refrigeration.

(B) 2 hours after receiving.

(C) 4 hours after refrigeration.

(D) 4 hours after receiving.

83) Which of the following is avoided by not rimming a clot from the sides of a tube?

(A) Hemolysis.

(B) Hemoconcentration.

(C) Hematoma.

(D) Blood-borne pathogen exposure.

84) How long can a prothrombin time specimen remain at room temperature?

(A) 2 hours.

(B) 4 hours.

(C) 8 hours.

(D) 24 hours.

85) How long can ESR specimens in EDTA tubes be refrigerated?

(A) 12 hours.

(B) 24 hours.

(C) 48 hours.

(D) 72 hours.

86) Which of the following categories of infectious substances do newborn screening cards belong to?

(A) Category A.

(B) Category B.

(C) Category C.

(D) Category D.

87) When you are receiving a 24-hour urine sample from a patient, he mentions that he forgot to collect a small amount when he went to urinate at night. You should do which of the following?

(A) Immediately refrigerate the specimen.

(B) Dilute the sample with a preservative.

(C) Ask the patient to submit a new one.

(D) Accept the specimen.

88) Your new colleague has forgotten his password to the LIS and is asking you to lend your password so he can print out requisition forms. You should do which of the following?

(A) Give him your password.

(B) Print out the requisition forms yourself.

(C) Give him your password, but immediately change it after he uses your account.

(D) All of the above.

89) Which of the following is the ideal temperature for storing serum or plasma, which cannot be tested after 48 hours?

(A) 27° C.

(B) 10° C.

(C) -20° C.

(D) 7° C.

90) Which of the following tests have a relatively lower risk of false results and no training requirement?

(A) Waived test.

(B) Provider-performed microscopy.

(C) Moderate complexity.

(D) High-complexity.

91) Performance of which of the following tests is subject to proficiency testing?

(A) Waived test.

(B) Provider-performed microscopy.

(C) High-complexity.

(D) Moderate-complexity.

92) Which of the following stipulates the standards that every laboratory must follow in the course of diagnostic procedures, professional qualifications, quality-management systems, and handling complaints?

(A) CLIA.

(B) HIPAA.

(C) OSHA.

(D) CAP.

93) Waived testing sites are not regularly inspected. Under which of the following circumstances will CMS inspect these sites?

(A) When a complaint has been raised.

(B) To ascertain whether these sites are performing only the tests they are permitted to.

(C) To gather data on waived tests.

(D) All of the above.

94) Certain situations may allow modifications of test kits for purposes other than what is intended. This is referred to as which of the following?

(A) Waived testing.

(B) Under-the-table testing.

(C) Off-label testing.

(D) Uncertified testing.

95) An external control determines which of the following?

(A) Whether a test is working properly.

(B) Whether the results fall within the expected range.

(C) Whether the sample size is adequate.

(D) All of the above.

96) When the results of a quality-control test are incorrect, which of the following is the most appropriate next step?

(A) Withhold reporting all patient test results from this batch.

(B) Complete the patient tests as these are timebound and cannot be withheld.

(C) Contact the manufacturer immediately and demand a refund.

(D) All of the above.

97) Which of the following statements is correct regarding waived testing?

(A) Swabs included in the test kits are interchangeable with sterile swabs.

(B) Only dermal puncture blood can be used on waived testing.

(C) Do not mark the test strips or cassettes.

(D) A phlebotomist may be assigned to perform a waived test.

98) When a result is invalid, which of the following is the next best step?

(A) Report the results now and repeat the test; report the repeated result.

(B) Do not report the results. Repeat the test and report both results.

(C) Do not report the results. Repeat the test and report only the repeated result.

(D) Do not report the results. Correct the problem. Repeat the test and report only the repeated result.

99) Which of the following are correct actions when reporting results over the telephone?

(A) Provide the results to any caller.

(B) Document the call and mark the copy of the test results as "reported."

(C) Document the call and promptly provide a written report.

(D) All of the above.

100) Whom among the following performs an internal quality assessment?

(A) Staff member.

(B) A consultant.

(C) Proficiency testing program.

(D) All of the above.

101) You are assigned to venipuncture for 12 patients in the ward. The patient in bed 8 does not wake up when you call his name. You should do which of the following first?

(A) Pinch the patient.

(B) Move on to the other patients.

(C) Perform a sternal rub.

(D) Inform the nurse, then move on to the other patients.

102) The depth of chest compressions in adults should be which of the following?

(A) 1.5 inches.

(B) 1.5 cm.

(C) 2 inches.

(D) 2 cm.

103) The rate of chest compressions should be which of the following?

(A) 100 to 120 per minute in adults.

(B) 100 to 120 per minute in children.

(C) 100 to 120 per minute in infants.

(D) All of the above.

104) Which of the following refers to how facilities adhere to laboratory standards, and evaluate the systems to prevent problems and resolve issues?

(A) Quality management.

(B) Quality assessment.

(C) Quality systems essentials.

(D) Quality control.

105) Which of the following organizations oversees quality-management systems?

(A) The Joint Commission.

(B) CLSI.

(C) CLIA.

(D) CAP.

106) Which of the following quality assessment documents provides a description of the principles and purpose for each test, specimen and collection requirements, a list of materials needed, special precautions (if any), procedure instructions, corrective actions, quality-control methods, and reference ranges?

(A) Procedural manuals.

(B) Policies.

(C) Reference manuals.

(D) Competency assessment.

107) A phlebotomist erroneously inserted a test report in the wrong patient's chart. This is an example of which of the following?

(A) Pre-examination variables.

(B) Examination variables.

(C) Post-examination variables.

(D) None of the above.

108) Which of the following is correct when documenting on the patient's chart?

(A) Use black ink.

(B) Utilize only standardized abbreviations.

(C) When correcting errors, strike it out with a single and sign your initials.

(D) All of the above.

109) Which of the following refers to the length of time that transpires from the moment a test is requisitioned up to the time results are generated and reported?

(A) Waiting period.

(B) Turnaround time.

(C) STAT.

(D) Lead-generation time.

110) The Lean system includes which of the following steps?

(A) Sorting, straightening, scrubbing, safety, standardizing, sustaining.

(B) Scrubbing, safety, standardizing, sustaining, sorting, straightening.

(C) Safety, sustaining, standardizing, straightening, scrubbing, sorting.

(D) Straightening, safety, scrubbing, sustaining, standardizing, sorting.

111) A misidentified patient has a hemolytic transfusion reaction. This is an example of which of the following?

(A) Sentinel event.

(B) Incident event.

(C) Critical event.

(D) Nonconforming events.

112) Which of the following documents is written by a witness and outlines the details of an incident and the actions taken to correct these?

(A) Sentinel event report.

(B) Incident report.

(C) Critical event report.

(D) Nonconforming events report.

113) Where can you find warning signs alerting you to corresponding transmission-based precautions for each patient?

(A) On the requisition form.

(B) In the patient charts.

(C) On the patient's ID bands.

(D) On the doors of patient rooms.

114) When a second venipuncture attempt is unsuccessful, which of the following is the most appropriate action?

(A) Attempt a third venipuncture on another site.

(B) Have the nurse perform the venipuncture.

(C) Notify the nurse and request another phlebotomist.

(D) Scold the patient for being uncooperative.

115) Which of the following is a hypertrophic scar resulting from excess collagen produced during skin healing?

(A) Keloid.

(B) Impetigo.

(C) Eczema.

(D) Dermatitis.

116) A phlebotomist is not allowed to remain at work until they are out of the infectious stage of all except which of the following diseases?

(A) Conjunctivitis.

(B) COVID-19.

(C) Acute gastroenteritis.

(D) Herpes zoster.

117) Which of the following pathogens commonly encountered in healthcare facilities is highly associated with antibiotic resistance?

(A) MRSA.

(B) Enterococcus.

(C) Clostridium difficile.

(D) All of the above.

118) Where are most releasing hormones produced?

(A) Endocrine organs.

(B) Hypothalamus.

(C) Anterior pituitary gland.

(D) Posterior pituitary gland.

119) Which of the following laboratory tests is paired with its correct clinical correlation?

(A) Amylase and infections.

(B) GGT and fat absorption.

(C) Sweat chloride test and cystic fibrosis.

(D) Cold agglutinin and organ failure.

120) Which of the following medical terms is used to refer to the outpouching of a blood vessel wall layer due to weakness?

(A) Aneurysm.

(B) Arteriosclerosis.

(C) Atherosclerosis.

(D) Embolism.

Test 1 Answers and Explanations

1) (C) Taking vital signs.

A phlebotomist may be assigned other tasks, including performing additional responsibilities related to patient care, such as taking vital signs.

2) (D) All of the above.

Communicating effectively involves listening, gestures, and an appropriate tone of voice.

3) (B) They extend their left arm.

Implied consent is commonly encountered with venipuncture. The patient implies consent when they allow you to proceed by extending or exposing their arm.

Nodding in agreement (C) is insufficient to imply consent in this case.

4) (B) Noticing the patient's reactions and accommodating them.

Being sensitive to cultural diversity is a desirable professional trait in the health care staff. A phlebotomist can respond appropriately by paying attention to the patient's reactions.

5) (D) HIPAA.

As outlined in HIPAA, all health care providers, including you as a phlebotomist, must obtain a patient's express consent in writing to share their information.

By releasing patient information to the patient's relatives or your fellow healthcare workers, or by inappropriately accessing electronic records, you can be charged with violating HIPAA. Consequences may range from suspension to imprisonment. You may even be charged with defamation for breaching a patient's confidentiality.

6) (C) Reservoir.

The chain of infection consists of six links. Take note from the scenarios that the susceptible host who contracts the disease becomes the new reservoir.

A newly-trained phlebotomist (susceptible host) sustains a needlestick from a patient (reservoir) with hepatitis B (infectious agent). He fails to report this incident. Unknowingly, he (the new reservoir) passes the infection to his girlfriend after unprotected intercourse (mode of transmission). In this case, he becomes the reservoir through which the hepatitis B virus is transmitted.

7) (B) Washing your hands.

Crucial moments for handwashing (recommended by the CDC):

- Before entering a patient's immediate environment
- Before carrying out an aseptic procedure, such as the insertion of an indwelling catheter (even when you will wear gloves)
- After leaving a patient's bed, room, or ward
- After handling bodily fluids (i.e., blood) or any contaminated surfaces
- After removing gloves

8) (A) The most contaminated items are removed first.

When removing PPE, the most contaminated items must be removed first. Make sure these do not contact your skin. The order for removing PPE is gloves first, then goggles or face shields, gown, and mask.

9) (B) Standard precautions.

This includes PPE, such as gloves, masks, gowns, etc. These precautions are used for all patients, even if they may not have an infection. This helps prevent the spread of pathogens from patient to patient.

10) (D) Sharp.

Sharps waste does not only refer to needles and blades. It includes metals or glass with edges that may cut or puncture.

11) (A) Waste bin.

PPEs usually consist of a mask, face protection, gown, and gloves. In a medical setting, PPE also includes a waste bin or a biohazard container. However, a waste bin is not donned.

12) (B) Connective.

Connective tissue provides a scaffold of support for the organs. The epithelial tissues (A) cover the lining of the body. The muscles (C) are specialized for movement. The nervous tissues (D) are specialized for impulse transmission.

13) (A) Nearer to the center of the body than the hand.

The directional term *proximal* was used, which describes the structure as nearer to the center of the body. Therefore, the elbow is nearer to the body's center than to the hand.

14) (A) Frontal.

The frontal plane cuts the body into anterior and posterior sections.

15) (C) Cranial.

Within the ventral cavity are the thoracic, abdominal, and pelvic subcavity.

16) (B) Carotid.

The carotid artery is often used to spot pulses during emergencies. It is a large artery branching near the aorta, while the rest of the choices are veins.

17) (A) Disseminated intravascular coagulation.

Pathogens and the inflammatory reaction during sepsis may trigger the coagulation process to ensue throughout the body, resulting in disseminated intravascular coagulation.

18) (A) The neck, elbow crease, and wrists.

When you are feeling someone's pulse, you are feeling the rhythmic waves that travel through the arteries from the pumping heart. Common areas to locate the pulse are the neck (carotid artery), the anterior elbow crease (brachial artery), and the wrist (radial artery).

19) (B) Neutrophils.

These types of leukocytes make up an average of 40% to 60% of all leukocytes found in the human body.

20) (A) Phlebitis.

Phlebitis is a condition that phlebotomists can inflict if they are not being careful. This refers to pain and swelling of the vein. An indwelling IV cannula can also be the culprit of this condition.

21) (B) Prothrombin time.

The prothrombin time can estimate the function of the extrinsic pathway and is useful in monitoring the response to warfarin therapy.

22) (A) Systolic blood pressure.

Blood pressure determines the pressure on the blood vessel walls during systole and diastole. It is measured in millimeters of mercury and reported as two numbers. The one above is the systole, while the one below is the diastole. This is normally at 120/80 mmHg for adults.

23) (C) Pulmonary artery.

The pulmonary artery is the only artery carrying deoxygenated blood. It gains the name "artery" because, like all the other arteries, it carries blood away from the heart.

24) (C) Urine cups.

Routine equipment seen on a phlebotomist's tray includes materials for the ETS (A), syringes (D), winged collection set, tourniquets (B), antiseptic skin solutions, gloves, gauze, slides, markers, transfer devices, and a sharps disposal container. The phlebotomist is not expected to carry urine collection cups.

25) (B) Binding calcium.

Anticoagulants prevent blood clot formation by binding calcium (ethylenediaminetetraacetic acid) or inhibiting thrombin (heparin).

26) (B) Green.

Anticoagulants prevent the formation of blood clots. Tubes containing heparin include green, light-green, lime-green, royal-blue, and red/green cell preparation tubes.

27) (B) Na fluoride.

Sodium fluoride prevents glycolysis and stabilizes glucose for 24 hours.

28) (D) All of the above.

Venipuncture begins when a phlebotomist receives the requisition form. It may be brought in by a patient from their doctor's clinic, received through the pneumatic tube, or electronically encoded in the hospital information system.

29) (B) Ask every patient to verbally state their first and last names and birth date.

CLSI standards require two identifiers. Ask every patient to verbally state their first and last names, spell them out, and give their birth date. Compare these to the data written on their ID bands with the requisition forms.

30) (C) Draw the blood as instructed and make sure to note "not fasting" on the requisition form.

Verify special preparations. These include appropriate fasting and skipping medications. In cases when the patient has not complied, report it to the nurse. If the nurse informs you that the physician still requires the specimen, document it on the requisition form and the specimen label as "not fasting."

31) (B) A 24-year-old undergoing chemotherapy.

The winged collection set, or "butterfly" system, is routinely used for IV infusions and venipuncture in smaller and very fragile veins. These are often encountered in cancer patients, small children, and geriatric patients.

32) (A) Winged collection system.

Small superficial veins are also found on the dorsum of the hand. These may be suitable for venipuncture. Smaller needles or butterfly sets are used to collect blood from this area. Often, this area is reserved for IV lines.

33) (B) 120 seconds.

The tourniquet should be used only for a maximum of 1 minute. You will often apply the tourniquet twice. First, choose the venipuncture site, and second, right before you draw blood. CLSI recommends waiting for at least 2 minutes before reapplying the tourniquet. Ideally, one new disposable, latex-free tourniquet is used for one patient. This avoids BBP and microbial transmission.

34) (C) At least 3 or 4 inches superior to the antecubital fossa.

To properly apply the tourniquet, choose a site on the arm at least 3 or 4 inches superior to the antecubital fossa. The tourniquet should be applied to a muscle.

35) (B) Hemoconcentration.

Pumping the fists causes hemoconcentration. This action is ideal for blood donation but not for laboratory testing.

36) (B) Instruct the patient to open their fist.

During a successful venipuncture, instruct the patient to open their fist as soon as the blood starts flowing down the tube. The tourniquet is released only if the procedure takes more than 1 minute.

37) (C) Hematoma.

Ensure the needle is removed from the vein before applying any pressure to the site. Keep pressure on the site. Or, if the patient is capable, ask them to hold down the gauze for about 2 to 3 minutes. Bending the elbow is not advisable, as it does not provide enough pressure. This causes blood to leak into the tissues, contributing to a hematoma.

38) (A) Patient ID number.

The specimen label must contain the following information:

- Patient identifiers: first name and last name
- Patient ID number (admitted patients) or birth date (for outpatient)
- Your initials as the phlebotomist
- Date and time collected

39) (D) Bilirubin is photosensitive; the tube must be wrapped in foil during transport.

Photosensitive analytes deteriorate upon exposure to light or ultraviolet radiation. These specimens may be wrapped in aluminum foil or collected in amber-colored tubes.

Choice A: Glycolysis falsely decreases glucose levels.

Choice B: Hemolysis falsely increases potassium levels

Choice C: Coagulation factors may be labile to temperature.

40) (D) Find the nurse to attach an ID band to the patient.

All admitted patients should have an ID band. If the band is missing, the correct action should be to find the nurse to replace the bands before you draw the blood.

A nurse may be allowed to sign the requisition slip to verify the patient's identity, but you still need to compare the patient's ID band with the requisition form.

41) (C) Cognitively impaired.

For patients who are too young, have cognitive impairments, or do not speak English, CLSI requires patient information to be provided by a caregiver. In some instances, the nurse may verify the patient's identity. You must document the informant's name on the requisition form.

42) (B) The patient is well-rested and fasted.

It is preferable to obtain specimens during the basal state. This is when the patient is well-rested and fasting (no food or drinks except water for the last 12 hours). This is often early in the morning. Venipuncture during the basal state achieves the best comparison of patient test values with reference ranges.

43) (B) Patients should lie down for 30 minutes before drawing blood for aldosterone tests.

Values for renin and aldosterone, and catecholamines can increase to twice their original values in an hour after shifting positions. For such tests, patients are instructed to stay recumbent for at least 30 minutes before blood is drawn. Additionally, you must note down on the requisition forms the patient's position during venipuncture.

44) (A) Remove the tourniquet and needle, apply pressure to the site, and summon help.

While it is rare, venipuncture may trigger seizures. When a patient suddenly starts having jerky movements and is unresponsive, immediately release the tourniquet and withdraw the needle. Apply pressure to the venipuncture site. While doing this, call for help. Make sure the patient is safe from possible injuries. Turn their head to one side. Do not attempt to place any object in their mouth. Do not leave the patient.

45) (A) Performing venipuncture on sclerotic veins.

Hemoconcentration affects many test results. It can be caused by venipuncture on sclerotic veins or edematous limbs.

46) (A) Below a hematoma.

Do not perform venipuncture in areas with possible infections, contamination, or low blood flow. Avoid venipuncture over hematomas, on edematous limbs, on sclerosed veins, or on burns, scars, or a new tattoo. When no other veins are suitable except for one near a hematoma, always puncture inferior to the hematoma. This ensures a sample of circulating blood.

47) (C) Collect blood from the other arm.

Patients undergoing hemodialysis often have a venous access device. It is more prone to infection and prolonged bleeding. Only trained staff can draw blood from these areas. You must first be sure that the arm has no grafts or fistulas before you apply a tourniquet. Compressing the vessels of these arms can compromise the integrity of these devices. Draw blood only on the arm without an arteriovenous graft or fistula.

48) (B) Needle advanced too deep into the vein.

When using the ETS, you must firmly brace the holder as you insert or change the tubes. If you fail to do so, the needle may puncture too deep into the vein. This goes through the vein and into the tissues. This obstructs blood flow and creates a hematoma. Slowly pulling the needle may remedy this situation. Be sure to apply additional pressure on the puncture site to reduce the risk of hematoma.

49) (C) Using a large needle on a small vein.

Technical errors leading to hematoma formation include:

- Forgetting to release the tourniquet before withdrawing the needle
- Applying inadequate pressure to the site
- Bending the patient's elbow over the site
- Improper probing
- Improper needle insertion technique
- Using a large needle on a small vein
- Puncturing the brachial artery

50) (D) Clotted lavender tubes.

Instances when a specimen is rejected include:

- No labels or improper labels
- Underfilled tubes
- Using the wrong tubes
- Hemolyzed samples
- Lipemic samples
- Presence of clots in an anticoagulated tube
- Improper handling, such as not covering a light-sensitive specimen
- Contaminated containers
- Delayed transport
- Using an expired tube
- Specimen with no requisition form

Lavender tubes contain EDTA as an anticoagulant. They should be inverted 8 times to ensure proper mixing. A clotted lavender tube will be rejected.

51) (D) All of the above.

Instances when adults require a dermal puncture include all of the above (chemotherapy patients, elderly, and those on glucose monitoring) as well as burn patients, and those with scarred and inaccessible veins (i.e., thrombosed, obesity).

52) (D) Newborn screening test.

Newborn screening tests use a specialized filter paper (Guthrie card), which relies on blood collected from a dermal puncture. Using capillary pipettes and other methods causes scratches and blood layering, which interferes with the integrity of the sample. A dermal puncture cannot provide adequate blood volume to run tests requiring larger volumes, such as coagulation assays, ESR, and blood cultures.

53) (C) Glucose.

Analytes from capillary blood may require a different set of reference values. It contains higher glucose levels and lower potassium, calcium, and protein levels than venous blood.

54) (B) Cause blood to collect and flow in the grooves.

In performing finger punctures, the device's blade is aligned across the grooves of the skin to create a perpendicular cut. This allows you to collect most of the blood, as it does not flow into these grooves.

55) (C) Make a note of agitation and crying in the requisition form.

Agitation and crying may affect white cell counts and blood glucose levels. Make a note of this on the requisition form.

56) (B) It increases blood flow.

Warming the fingers and heels increases blood circulation, which eases specimen collection. This is optimal for collecting multiple samples, capillary blood glucose sampling, and cold and cyanotic areas.

57) (A) It avoids contamination.

Wipe off the initial drop of blood using a gauze unless the tests require otherwise. This practice avoids collecting samples contaminated with residual alcohol or tissue fluids.

58) (B) Galactosemia.

Galactosemia is due to the lack of an enzyme that normally metabolizes galactose, which is found in milk. This accumulates in the blood and causes problems in multiple organs, such as the liver, brain, and kidneys. The damage is prevented by placing these infants on a lactose-free and galactose-free diet.

59) (A) Using one drop of blood from a heel puncture to fill and soak one circle.

The blood from the heel puncture is blotted on an area marked by circles on the specimen card. To ensure the sample's integrity, you must avoid contaminating this area with other chemicals or even your fingerprints. Use only one drop of blood on each circle, and apply each to the same side. Do not touch the paper to the infant's heel. An adequate sample is also visible on the back side of the card. Each circle must be adequately filled.

60) (A) On the feathered edge.

A properly prepared smear has a smooth film covering about 2/3 of the slide without any creases or holes. It ends smoothly, as a feathered edge. This area ensures that the cells are spread in a single even layer. The feathered edge is the area viewed under the microscope to ensure that the reading is looking at a sample representative of the patient's blood.

61) (A) Sepsis.

Sepsis is the clinical term used when the patient has a systemic inflammation (such as fever and increased heart rate, or increased white cell counts), along with bacteremia, or the presence of bacteria in the bloodstream.

62) (B) Just before the height of fever.

The blood culture is usually collected as two sets of blood taken 30 minutes or 1 hour apart. Some physicians may request the cultures to be collected just before the height of the fever (based on the patterns in the temperature charts) to collect the most concentration of pathogens.

63) (B) Collect the sample in special bottles containing activated charcoal.

Special blood culture bottles are available when it is necessary to take a blood culture sample from patients already taking antibiotics. These may contain resins (antimicrobial removal devices) or activated charcoal (fastidious antimicrobial neutralization) designed to inactivate antibiotics.

64) (B) 70% isopropyl alcohol.

Chlorhexidine gluconate is not suitable for use on infants below 2 months old. It is highly irritating to their sensitive skin and can possibly cause chemical burns. ChloraPrep swabs contain a mixture of chlorhexidine gluconate and alcohol. Of the choices, only 70% isopropyl alcohol is adequate and safe for cleansing the skin of a newborn.

65) (C) 1 mL in only one pediatric bottle.

Pediatric bottles are available for use on children. The volume of blood collected is computed based on the child's weight. From an infant weighing less than 5 kg, collect only 1 ml in one bottle.

66) (B) Serum potassium.

Chilling is not suitable for testing some analytes. Potassium increases in a chilled tube. Electrolyte tests must be collected separately when drawing blood with chilling requirements.

67) (C) You should document your name and the date and time on the chain-of-custody form.

Specimen handling is documented extensively when collecting forensic samples for legal proceedings. Each person involved in the chain of custody must document their name and the date and time they handled the specimen.

68) (B) Underfilling the gray tube.

Alcohol is a volatile substance and may escape into the surrounding air. Gray tubes (with sodium fluoride) must be filled until the vacuum is exhausted. They must remain covered until testing. Underfilling allows alcohol to escape in the surrounding air left in the tube, causing falsely low blood alcohol levels.

69) (D) Hemoglobin count of 13 g/dL.

The eligibility criteria for blood donation allow a 16-year-old (A) to donate only with consent from their parents or guardians. Volunteers should weigh at least 50 kg (B), be afebrile, with normal blood pressure below 180/100 mmHg (C), with hemoglobin of ≥ 12.5 g/dL (D), and hematocrit of ≥ 38%.

70) (D) All of the above.

Donor screening also involves testing a sample of the blood for ABO and Rh blood type and testing for the presence of blood-borne pathogens. Donor units are tested for parasites, such as *Trypanosoma cruzi*, and viruses, such as HIV, hepatitis B and C, HTLV, and West Nile virus. Testing for *Treponema pallidum* is also done.

71) (A) 16- or 17-gauge.

A large-gauge needle (16- or 17-gauge) is necessary to prevent hemolysis and allow large volumes to be collected.

72) (A) Autologous donation.

Of the choices, only (A) is correct. Patients who need elective surgery may preemptively donate a unit of their blood to be transfused during or after their operation. An autologous donation avoids transfusion reactions and exposure to bloodborne pathogens.

73) (D) Return to work involving lifting heavy objects.

A significant amount of blood has been removed during the blood collection. Donors should replenish their fluids by drinking plenty of fluids and avoid complications by refraining from strenuous activities or heavy lifting during the day. They cannot be allowed to return to work involving lifting heavy objects, as this might cause them to faint from the strain.

74) (A) Catheter collection.

For bacterial cultures, especially on bedridden patients or infants, trained personnel collect a sample by passing a sterile catheter into the patient's urethra under aseptic conditions.

75) (A) Immersing the swab in saline and mixing it vigorously.

For nasopharyngeal swabs, after collection, it is immersed and mixed in a saline transport medium vigorously. Any excess liquid should be squeezed out of the swab before disposing of it. The tube, not the swab, is transported on an ice slurry.

76) (C) Tubes may be used to transport specimens collected through invasive means.

A pneumatic tube system is available in many hospitals to facilitate the delivery of specimens from the wards to the laboratory. Tubes must be properly cushioned and kept in leak-proof biohazard containers. Specimens collected through invasive means must be transported only by hand. This avoids any untoward incidents from a pneumatic tube transit.

77) (B) Synovial fluid.

Synovial fluid is also known as joint fluids. This acts as a lubricant during movement.

78) (D) All of the above.

CSF is collected in three sterile tubes labeled according to the order of collection. The first tube is intended for chemistry and immunoserology assays. The second tube is for microbiology, and the third is for hematology and cytology.

79) (D) Peritoneal.

Peritoneal fluid is found between the membranes of the abdominal cavity. An increase in the peritoneal fluid is also known as ascites.

80) (B) Hydrogen breath test.

Increasing levels of hydrogen in breath indicate malabsorption or indigestion of lactose in the gastrointestinal tract, which may aid in the diagnosis of lactose intolerance.

81) (A) Do not eat or drink.

The first-morning sample is ideal to ensure a large enough collection. Patients are instructed to collect the samples before a meal and without smoking. Moments before the expectoration of sputum, have the patient gargle with water (but do not swallow) to obtain a sample with the least contamination.

82) (B) 2 hours after receiving.

Centrifugation must be completed within 2 hours of receiving the specimen to avoid analyte changes.

83) (A) Hemolysis.

Do not rim a clotted tube. This can lead to hemolysis.

84) (D) 24 hours.

Prothrombin time specimen may remain at room temperature for up to 24 hours. Chilling is not recommended, as it can activate factor VII.

85) (A) 12 hours.

Erythrocyte sedimentation rates should be analyzed from 4 hours of collection in EDTA tubes kept at room temperature. Refrigeration may extend this limit by up to 12 hours.

86) (B) Category B.

Biohazardous material may be designated one of two classifications. Most laboratory specimens fall in category B—not generally disabling or life-threatening to humans or animals.

87) (C) Ask the patient to submit a new one.

A 24-hour urine collection is used to provide a quantitative measure of urine analytes. In this situation, you should politely reject the specimen and remind the patient of the importance of collecting all the samples to keep the results accurate.

88) (B) Print out the requisition forms yourself.

In this case, the best option would be to print out the requisition forms yourself since you would be accountable for any mistakes your colleague may make. Never share your password with anyone. All data within the LIS may be traced back to who has inputted it or handled the specimen.

89) (C) -20° C.

Freezing may be done if testing is expected to be done beyond 48 hours. This is achieved at temperatures -20° C or lower.

90) (A) Waived test.

These diagnostic procedures are simple. No training is required. There is little to no risk of error when following the box instructions.

91) (C) High-complexity.

These procedures utilize complex instrumentation. Interpretation requires higher levels of understanding, and the performance of these tests is subject to proficiency testing.

92) (A) CLIA.

CLIA stipulates the standards that every laboratory must follow in diagnostic procedures, professional qualifications, quality-management systems, and handling complaints. These are set by the Center for Medicare & Medicaid Services (CMS).

93) (D) All of the above.

Certain circumstances when CMS will include inspection of waived testing procedures during its surveillance at dedicated testing sites include:

- When a complaint has been raised
- To ascertain whether these sites are performing only tests they are permitted to (i.e., certified waived tests)
- To gather data on waived tests

94) (C) Off-label testing.

Certain situations may allow modifications of test kits for purposes other than what is written in the manufacturer's instructions. This means that the FDA did not clear the test kit for this off-label purpose or the manufacturer did not have enough data to support this.

95) (B) Whether the results fall within the expected range.

An external control determines whether a test is performed properly and whether the results fall within the expected range. External controls are provided by the manufacturer and appear like test samples.

96) (A) Withhold reporting all patient test results from this batch.

When the quality-control results are incorrect, all patient test results should be withheld until the problem has been identified and addressed.

97) (D) A phlebotomist may be assigned to perform a waived test.

After proper training, a phlebotomist may be assigned to perform waived testing.

Option A: Swabs included in the test kits are not interchangeable with sterile swabs. The differences in the material may provide inaccurate results.

Option B: Whole blood for waived tests may be collected through dermal puncture or venipuncture.

Option C: For test kits that require direct application of the sample onto the test device (strip or cassette).

98) (D) Do not report the results. Correct the problem. Repeat the test and report only the repeated result.

When results are invalid, do not report the results. Identify and address the problem first. Then, repeat all patient samples and report the corrected results.

99) (C) Document the call and promptly provide a written report.

When reporting a result verbally (such as over the telephone), document this and promptly provide a written report. Take note: provide copies of test reports only to the patient or an authorized person.

100) (A) staff member.

An internal assessment involves processes for the staff to self-evaluate their current performance and practices. This method involves performing quality control, reviewing these along with the test results, evaluating record-keeping practices, documenting issues, and creating an action plan to improve.

101) (A) Pinch the patient.

When you meet each patient, you should rouse them from sleep. Patients who have been arrested may just seem peacefully asleep. Therefore, if it is difficult to rouse a patient, try stimulating them with a loud noise, shaking them, or pinching their earlobe first. If they do not respond, elicit pain by performing a sternal rub. Do not simply walk away from this situation; the patient may have already been arrested, and you may have missed the opportunity to initiate life-saving cardiopulmonary responses before it is too late.

102) (C) 2 inches.

To perform chest compressions in adults, place both hands interlaced on the patient's lower sternum. Using the heel of one hand, push on the sternum to depress it at least 2 inches.

103) (D) All of the above.

The rate for chest compressions should be in the range of 100 to 120 per minute. This does not change in children, infants, or adults.

104) (A) Quality management.

Quality management refers to how a facility adheres to laboratory standards and evaluates the systems to prevent problems and resolve issues. It encompasses quality assessment and quality control.

105) (A) The Joint Commission.

This commission takes charge of accrediting healthcare institutions across the United States, intending to continually improve healthcare quality. Every two years, a survey team visits laboratories to assess their adherence to the National Patient Safety Goals and renews their accreditation. It oversees the quality-management systems of each facility.

106) (A) Procedural manuals.

Procedural manuals provide a description of the principles and purpose for each test, specimen, and collection requirements; a list of materials needed; special precautions (if any); procedure instructions; corrective actions; quality-control methods; and reference ranges.

107) (C) Post-examination variables.

Post-examination variables include all activities directed toward reporting test results to the patient or physician. This may be accomplished either by telephone, fax, or electronic mail.

108) (D) All of the above.

Guidelines for documenting in a patient's chart:

- Use black ink.
- Sign your initials with the date and time of collection.
- Utilize only standardized abbreviations (when necessary).
- Write complete documentation of your actions as well as patient actions.
- To correct an error on paper, draw a single line across it and sign your initials.
- To correct an error online, do not erase the previous entry; instead, enter the updated result with a comment alerting you to the new entry.

109) (B) Turnaround time.

This refers to the time that transpires from when a test is requisitioned to when its results are generated and reported. This is determined by each facility.

110) (A) Sorting, straightening, scrubbing, safety, standardizing, sustaining.

The Lean system involves six steps:

1. Sorting
2. Straightening
3. Scrubbing
4. Safety
5. Standardizing
6. Sustaining

111) (A) Sentinel event.

A sentinel event refers to an unexpected severe injury, often leading to death in the context of health care provision.

112) (B) Incident report.

The incident report allows a witness to describe an incident and the actions taken to correct it. This documents and investigates the incident.

113) (D) On the doors of patient rooms.

On the doors of patient rooms, warning signs may be posted to alert you to transmission-based precautions and the corresponding PPE for these patients.

114) (C) Notify the nurse and request another phlebotomist.

When a second venipuncture attempt is unsuccessful, do not try a third. Notify the nurse and request another phlebotomist to collect the specimen.

115) (A) Keloid.

Keloid is a type of hypertrophic scar resulting from excess collagen produced during skin healing.

116) (C) Acute gastroenteritis.

Acute gastroenteritis is not communicable. The following are common communicable diseases. A phlebotomist is not allowed to remain at work until they are out of the infectious stage:

- Active hepatitis A
- Active tuberculosis
- Bacterial or viral conjunctivitis
- COVID-19 (even if asymptomatic or mild)
- Dysentery
- Flu or influenza
- Herpes zoster
- Infection with lice or scabies
- Measles
- Mumps
- Pertussis
- Streptococcal tonsilitis
- Varicella

117) (D) All of the above.

Common pathogens associated with antibiotic resistance encountered in healthcare facilities include methicillin-resistant *staphylococcus aureus*, *enterococcus*, and *clostridium difficile.*

118) (B) Hypothalamus.

The hypothalamus is responsible for producing and secreting releasing hormones.

119) (C) Sweat chloride test and cystic fibrosis.

Only Option C is correct.

120) (A) Aneurysm.

Aneurysm is the outpouching of a blood vessel wall layer due to weakness. It is a serious condition, as it may progress, increase in size, or burst, leading to a hemorrhage.

Test 2 Questions

1) As a phlebotomist, you can display professional behavior in the facility by doing which of the following?

(A) Keeping your workstation neat and organized.

(B) Wearing a lot of cologne.

(C) Slouching and not maintaining eye contact when you enter the patient's room.

(D) Wearing a dirty lab coat .

2) A phlebotomist can display empathy and make patients feel reassured by doing which of the following?

(A) Taking a phone call during the procedure.

(B) Avoiding eye contact.

(C) Crossing their arms.

(D) Walking tall as they enter a patient's room.

3) Which statement is correct regarding procedures in reverse isolation areas?

(A) When phlebotomy is completed, you must take all equipment out with you.

(B) In reverse isolation areas, all PPE must be sterile.

(C) Remove PPE only after leaving the room.

(D) All of the above.

4) A phlebotomist has not been trained with arterial blood extraction, but he proceeds to do so. The patient ends up with a nerve injury. The phlebotomist is committing which of the following?

(A) Negligence.

(B) Defamation.

(C) Malpractice.

(D) Assault.

5) Obtaining consent for HIV screening is which of the following?

(A) A requirement of the laws of your state.

(B) An opt-out procedure.

(C) An opt-in procedure.

(D) A service that requires express consent in writing.

6) The correct sequence of doffing PPE is which of the following?

(A) Gloves, goggles, mask, gown.

(B) Goggles, gloves, gown, mask.

(C) Mask, gloves, goggles, gown.

(D) Gloves, goggles, gown, mask.

7) Which of the following is not true of PPE in a medical setting as specified by OSHA?

(A) It is designed to limit exposure to hazardous material.

(B) It usually consists of a gown, facial protection, and gloves.

(C) It may include a waste bin or a biohazard container.

(D) It usually consists of hard hats and reflective gear.

8) Preventing transmission of pathogens includes which of the following precautions?

(A) Proper donning of personal protective equipment.

(B) Incomplete vaccinations.

(C) Reusing needles.

(D) Improper sharps disposal.

9) Blood-borne pathogens may be transmitted through which of the following exposure modes?

(A) Mucous membranes around the eyes.

(B) Intact skin.

(C) Properly sheathed needle.

(D) All of the above.

10) Alcohol disinfectant is not recommended in cases of contact with which organism?

(A) Clostridium botulinum.

(B) MRSA.

(C) Herpes simplex virus.

(D) Trichomonas vaginalis.

11) For healthcare workers, which of the following is not recommended?

(A) Having tattoos on either hand.

(B) Wearing jewelry.

(C) Wearing artificial nails.

(D) Having clean and short nails.

12) Which of the following precaution categories is employed to avoid respiratory hazards and infections, such as adenovirus, mumps, and tuberculosis?

(A) Emergency precautions.

(B) Standard precautions.

(C) Droplet precautions.

(D) Airborne precautions.

13) Contaminated equipment and used PPE and bandages belong to which of the following waste categories?

(A) Radioactive waste.

(B) Deadly waste.

(C) Biological waste.

(D) Exogenous material.

14) Body systems are made up of a few organs that coordinate to perform interrelated functions. One example of a body system is which of the following?

(A) Brain.

(B) Erythrocytes.

(C) Endocrine.

(D) Epithelium.

15) Which of the following planes cuts the body horizontally into upper and lower sections?

(A) Frontal.

(B) Sagittal.

(C) Midsagittal.

(D) Transverse.

16) Which of the following arteries is a common site for arterial blood extraction and may be located in the inguinal canal?

(A) Radial.

(B) Carotid.

(C) Brachial.

(D) Femoral.

17) Which of the following describes the correct way of determining an irregular pulse rate?

(A) Count the beats again for 5 minutes, then divide it by 5.

(B) Count the beats again for 30 seconds, then multiply by 2.

(C) Count the beats again for 1 full minute.

(D) Count the beats again for 2 full minutes.

18) How many liters of blood does the average human adult body contain?

(A) 0–1 liter.

(B) 2–3 liters.

(C) 4–5 liters.

(D) 5–6 liters.

19) It may or may not be present in the red blood cells. When a negative mother is sensitized by her fetus, the reaction is called the hemolytic disease of the newborn. Which of the following blood antigens is described?

(A) ABO.

(B) D antigen.

(C) RhD.

(D) anti-D.

20) When a monocyte is found in the lung tissues, it is often referred to as which of the following?

(A) Alveolar macrophage.

(B) Osteoclast.

(C) Microglia.

(D) Kupffer cell.

21) Which of the following stages of hemostasis is evaluated by a thrombin time?

(A) Primary.

(B) Secondary.

(C) Fibrin clot.

(D) Clot lysis.

22) Which of the following gives information on the time for one cardiac cycle to complete and the regularity of the cardiac rhythm?

(A) Pulse rate.

(B) Electrocardiogram.

(C) Blood pressure.

(D) Echocardiogram.

23) Which of the following kinds of blood vessels carry oxygenated blood?

(A) Pulmonary vein.

(B) Great saphenous vein.

(C) Pulmonary artery.

(D) Median cubital vein.

24) An expired collection tube causes which of the following problems?

(A) Short draw.

(B) Clotted serum samples.

(C) Completely filled tubes.

(D) None.

25) The phlebotomist should do which of the following before disposing of a used needle?

(A) Wipe the blood off.

(B) Recap the needle.

(C) Remove the needle from the ETS.

(D) Activate the needle's safety device.

26) Which of the following evacuated tubes is explicitly used for crossmatching samples?

(A) Lavender top.

(B) Red top.

(C) Pink top.

(D) Green top.

27) Which of the following kinds of information is not found on the requisition form?

(A) Patient ID number.

(B) The requesting physician's name and signature.

(C) Test(s) requested.

(D) Special handling requirements for the tests requested.

28) Before proceeding with a venipuncture, which of the following should be done?

(A) Use two identifiers to identify the correct patient.

(B) Obtain consent.

(C) Compare the patient's ID band with the requisition form.

(D) All of the above.

29) How should you position the patient's arm to facilitate proper venipuncture?

(A) Hyperextend the forearm.

(B) Position the arm so the wrist through the shoulder can be traced with a straight line.

(C) Bend the elbow at a 90° angle.

(D) Make sure the arms remain at the side, with the patient standing up.

30) Which of the following is important to consider when choosing the blood collection system?

(A) Patient's age.

(B) Blood volume to be extracted.

(C) Condition of the veins.

(D) All of thc above.

31) When both arms have no accessible median cubital veins, which of the following veins can be a second choice?

(A) Median cubital vein.

(B) Basilic vein.

(C) Cephalic vein.

(D) Axillary vein.

32) How long can a tourniquet be allowed to compress a vein?

(A) 60 seconds.

(B) 120 seconds.

(C) 180 seconds.

(D) 5 minutes.

33) How can a vein be properly palpated?

(A) Using the thumb.

(B) Using a tourniquet.

(C) Using the palms.

(D) Using the index finger.

34) To ensure the maximal bacteriostatic action of isopropyl alcohol, it is important to do which of the following?

(A) Wait for 1 minute for the alcohol to dry.

(B) Puncture the site while it is still wet.

(C) Fan the site to dry.

(D) Wipe the site with a cotton pad.

35) The angle of the needle for venipuncture should be which of the following?

(A) At a 15°- to 30°-angle with the bevel facing up.

(B) At a 45°- to 60°-angle with the bevel facing up.

(C) At a 15°- to 30°-angle with the bevel facing down.

(D) At a 45°- to 60°-angle with the bevel facing down.

36) The ideal time to invert the evacuated tubes with additives is which of the following?

(A) Immediately after it is removed from the ETS holder.

(B) On your way to the laboratory.

(C) When you have filled all tubes.

(D) While you label each specimen.

37) Which of the following is the maximum time to centrifuge a coagulation assay specimen after receiving it?

(A) 2 hours.

(B) 1 hour.

(C) 45 minutes.

(D) 30 minutes.

38) Before releasing an outpatient, the phlebotomist should do which of the following?

(A) Thank the patient.

(B) Bandage their arm.

(C) Remind them to eat if they have no other procedures.

(D) All of the above.

39) You must do which of the following before performing venipuncture in the outpatient setting?

(A) Read out the patient's name; check if they nod or say yes.

(B) Call out the patient's name from the waiting room and see who approaches you.

(C) Compare the patient's ID band with the requisition form.

(D) Verify their information with their photo ID card and see if these match the requisition slip.

40) You arrive at a patient's ward, but she is still sleeping. Which of the following actions is appropriate?

(A) Wake her gently, identify yourself, and wait for her to be oriented.

(B) Postpone the procedure; leave the requisition with the nurses.

(C) Wait for her family member.

(D) Find the nurse to wake her.

41) When encountering an unidentified patient in the emergency department, which of the following actions is recommended by the American Association of Blood Banks?

(A) Do not draw blood from these patients.

(B) Cross-reference their temporary ID number with their permanent number.

(C) Put a temporary ID band on the patient.

(D) Wait until their identity is confirmed before you can do venipuncture.

42) Why are most routine venipunctures often collected early in the morning?

(A) Physicians usually make rounds in the morning and need these results early.

(B) The patient is well-rested and fasted.

(C) The patient will have already had breakfast.

(D) Fewer adverse reactions (i.e., nausea, fainting) are encountered.

43) Pre-examination variables affect the integrity of the specimens and alter test results. Which of the following statements is correct?

(A) Alcohol intake increases blood testosterone levels.

(B) Prolonged fasting does not affect blood tests.

(C) Venipuncture may proceed regardless of the patient's position.

(D) In crying children, white cell count may be elevated.

44) Your patient appears pale, cold, and clammy while you are about to perform venipuncture. Which of the following adverse reactions may develop?

(A) Syncope.

(B) Prolonged bleeding.

(C) Hematoma.

(D) Allergies.

45) Hemoconcentration is produced by which of the following actions?

(A) Probing the needle vigorously.

(B) Removing the tourniquet before 1 minute.

(C) Asking the patient to clench their fist.

(D) Inverting the evacuated tubes.

46) Which of the following areas is suitable for venipuncture?

(A) Hematoma.

(B) Edematous limbs.

(C) Sclerosed veins.

(D) Hand veins.

47) When attempting venipuncture on obese patients, which of the following can make their veins more prominent?

(A) Using a bariatric tourniquet.

(B) Using a syringe system with a longer needle.

(C) Blind probing to locate a vein.

(D) Only A and B.

48) Which of the following needle positions fills the tube too slowly and causes a hematoma to form?

(A) Bevel too close to the vessel wall.

(B) Needle advanced too deep into the vein.

(C) Needle angle too narrow.

(D) Needle is not inside the vein.

49) When a patient complains of tingling, shock-like sensations, overt pain, or numbness in the area, you suspect which of the following?

(A) Arterial injury.

(B) Nerve damage.

(C) Syncope.

(D) Vein collapse.

50) Which of the following technical errors leads to hemolysis?

(A) Inserting the needle through the vein.

(B) Using a 21-gauge needle.

(C) Drawing blood below a hematoma.

(D) Drawing blood from a sclerosed vein.

51) Dermal punctures would be inappropriate in which of the following instances?

(A) Severely dehydrated patients.

(B) Patients with edematous fingers.

(C) Blood culture test.

(D) All of the above.

52) Which of the following statements is correct?

(A) Capillary blood and venipuncture samples use the same set of reference values.

(B) Dermal puncture collects fluid from the tissues as well.

(C) Milking the area during a dermal puncture increases blood circulation.

(D) Cooling the site increases blood circulation.

53) The most important factor to consider in choosing a dermal puncture device is which of the following?

(A) Number of drops of blood needed.

(B) Depth of the puncture.

(C) Width of the incision.

(D) The blood volume needed.

54) On which of the following sites can a dermal puncture be safely performed?

(A) Third or fourth finger.

(B) Index finger.

(C) Toes.

(D) Back of the heel.

55) A phlebotomist performing dermal puncture can cause infections in the patient by doing which of the following?

(A) Accidentally puncturing the bone.

(B) Repeating the puncture on a previous site.

(C) Reusing a lancet.

(D) All of the above.

56) Which of the following happens when a dermal puncture is performed while alcohol is still wet?

(A) It can cause microclots.

(B) It causes platelet aggregation.

(C) It prevents the formation of a round drop of blood.

(D) It is soothing for the patient.

57) Which of the following is the correct order of draw for the following tests on dermal puncture: malarial smear, complete blood count, and bilirubin?

(A) Blood smears, complete blood count, bilirubin.

(B) Complete blood count, bilirubin, blood smears.

(C) Blood smears, bilirubin, complete blood count.

(D) Bilirubin, blood smears, complete blood count.

58) Which of the following is the best time to perform a newborn screening test?

(A) 24 hours after birth.

(B) 48 hours after discharge.

(C) 1 week after birth.

(D) 1 month after birth.

59) Which of the following is the ideal angle of the spreader slide when preparing a thin blood smear?

(A) 5 degrees.

(B) 15 degrees.

(C) 30 degrees.

(D) 45 degrees.

60) Which of the following is the use of a thick smear?

(A) To concentrate the sample to find and detect malarial parasites.

(B) To identify the morphology of malarial parasites.

(C) To prevent transmission of blood-borne pathogens.

(D) To use as a medium to grow parasites.

61) Which of the following tests is ordered to identify and detect pathogens causing bacteremia?

(A) Blood culture.

(B) Complete blood count.

(C) Thick blood smear.

(D) Lumbar puncture.

62) When no blood culture bottles are available, how should you collect the specimen?

(A) Postpone the test as it cannot be performed without the equipment.

(B) Use sterile yellow (SPS) evacuated tubes.

(C) Use sterile yellow (ACD) evacuated tubes.

(D) Use sterile red (plain) evacuated tubes.

63) Which of the following is true when you are using a winged (butterfly) collection system?

(A) The anaerobic bottle is filled first.

(B) The aerobic bottle is filled first.

(C) The volume of the blood collected is increased.

(D) Either bottle can be filled first.

64) To ensure adequate asepsis with a ChloraPrep swab, how long must you wait before venipuncture?

(A) 30 seconds.

(B) 1 minute.

(C) 2 minutes.

(D) It is not necessary to wait.

65) Why are blood volume requirements important to blood culture collection?

(A) To collect the least amount of blood while maintaining the proper blood-to-culture medium ratio.

(B) To prevent contamination of the sample with tissue fluid.

(C) To ensure adequate concentration of bacteria is collected.

(D) To prevent iatrogenic anemia.

66) Which of the following tests should be kept chilled?

(A) Arterial blood gases to be tested in 30 minutes.

(B) Ammonia.

(C) Cold agglutinin.

(D) Bilirubin.

67) Which of the following tests should be collected in amber-colored bottles?

(A) Porphyrins.

(B) Potassium.

(C) Glucose.

(D) Phosphorus.

68) Which of the following tests may be collected in a yellow (ACD) tube?

(A) Paternity testing samples.

(B) Blood alcohol testing.

(C) Blood cultures.

(D) Ammonia.

69) Which of the following characteristics would make a volunteer not eligible to donate blood?

(A) They received a vaccine for varicella 2 days ago.

(B) They took the last antibiotic pill for a complete course a few hours ago.

(C) They previously donated blood 10 weeks ago.

(D) They inject insulin before every meal.

70) Which of the following additives should be present in a blood bag to preserve the blood and prevent clots?

(A) Sodium polyanethol sulfonate.

(B) Citrate-phosphate-dextrose.

(C) Acid citrate dextrose.

(D) Ethylenediaminetetraacetic acid.

71) During the donor blood collection, which of the following actions is appropriate for the donor?

(A) Pump their fist to allow hemoconcentration of the blood.

(B) Shake their hands for a faster blood flow.

(C) Elevate their hands above their head for faster blood flow.

(D) Stand for the duration of the collection.

72) You are the receiving phlebotomist when you notice that a urine sample was collected over 2 hours before being delivered to the laboratory. You should do which of the following?

(A) Immediately refrigerate the specimen.

(B) Dilute the sample with a preservative.

(C) Ask the patient to submit a new one.

(D) Accept the specimen.

73) In performing a urine drug test, which of the following indicates urine sample tampering?

(A) pH of 9.5.

(B) The specific gravity of 1.005.

(C) Temperature is between 32.5ºC and 37.7ºC.

(D) All of the above.

74) Which of the following is an appropriate instruction for semen collection?

(A) Refrain from sexual activity for 3 days.

(B) Collect the sample in a sterile cup.

(C) Keep the sample warm.

(D) All of the above.

75) Nasopharyngeal swabs are requested for the detection of which of the following organisms?

(A) SARSCOV-2.

(B) RSV.

(C) Parainfluenza virus.

(D) All of the above.

76) Which of the following needles is used for bone marrow aspiration?

(A) 23-gauge needle.

(B) Large-bone, thin-diameter needle.

(C) Jamshidi needle.

(D) Guthrie needle.

77) Which of the following specimens may be used to investigate the organisms responsible for meningitis and other neurological pathologies?

(A) Amniotic fluid.

(B) Synovial fluid.

(C) Cerebrospinal fluid.

(D) Serous fluid.

78) Which of the following CSF tube numbers is correctly paired with its intended department?

(A) Tube 1 for hematology.

(B) Tube 2 for microbiology.

(C) Tube 3 for chemistry.

(D) All of the above.

79) Which of the following anticoagulants is appropriate for microbiologic cultures of synovial fluid?

(A) Heparin.

(B) EDTA.

(C) Sodium fluoride.

(D) None.

80) Ascites refers to the increase in which of the following serous fluids?

(A) Pleural.

(B) Pericardial.

(C) Parietal.

(D) Peritoneal.

81) *Helicobacter pylori* can be detected in the breath through which of the following tests?

(A) C-urea breath test.

(B) Hydrogen breath test.

(C) Alcohol breath test.

(D) Carbon dioxide breath test.

82) Which of the following is the default setting for centrifugation?

(A) 850 to 1,000 gravity for 10 minutes.

(B) 850 to 1,000 gravity for 20 minutes.

(C) 250 to 500 gravity for 10 minutes.

(D) 250 to 500 gravity for 20 minutes.

83) Which of the following is obtained after centrifugation of anticoagulated blood?

(A) Serum.

(B) Plasma.

(C) Buffy coat.

(D) Aliquot.

84) Which of the following statements is true regarding centrifugation?

(A) Keep all tubes closed and balance the rotor equally.

(B) Keep the centrifuge covered when operating.

(C) Observe the centrifuge for any excessive vibration before leaving the area.

(D) All of the above.

85) For how long can serum or plasma be adequately kept in a refrigerator?

(A) 8 hours.

(B) 24 hours.

(C) 48 hours.

(D) 72 hours.

86) For how long can CBC in EDTA microtainers remain at room temperature?

(A) 2 hours.

(B) 4 hours.

(C) 8 hours.

(D) 24 hours.

87) Which of the following categories of infectious substances is correctly paired?

(A) Category A is life-threatening only to animals.

(B) Category B is life-threatening to humans and animals.

(C) Category A is generally not life-threatening.

(D) Category B is generally not life-threatening.

88) When shipping laboratory specimens, how should the containers be marked?

(A) UN 2814 Biological Substance Category A.

(B) UN 3373 Biological Substance Category B.

(C) Class 9 miscellaneous.

(D) Class 10 miscellaneous.

89) The Laboratory Information Systems is capable of which of the following functions?

(A) Identifying the patient.

(B) Automatically informing the nurse and physicians of patient complications.

(C) Storing archive of a patient's health records.

(D) All of the above.

90) Which of the following tests requires training, an understanding of the principles, and knowledge of instrument calibration?

(A) Waived test.

(B) Provider-performed microscopy.

(C) Moderate complexity.

(D) High complexity.

91) Which of the following is a moderate complexity test?

(A) Urine pregnancy test.

(B) Glycosylated hemoglobin test.

(C) Capillary blood glucose.

(D) All of the above.

92) CMS may perform inspections and evaluate phlebotomists' performance in accordance with which of the following standards?

(A) CLIA.

(B) HIPAA.

(C) OSHA.

(D) CAP.

93) Waived testing sites are not regularly inspected. Under which of the following circumstances will CMS inspect these sites?

(A) To conduct proficiency testing.

(B) To scout for phlebotomists to be promoted to a moderate complexity site.

(C) To gather data on waived tests.

(D) All of the above.

94) A patient with anemia requires blood glucose testing. You use a glucometer on capillary blood despite the manufacturer's instructions to test only on patients with normal-range hematocrit. This is referred to as which of the following?

(A) Negligence.

(B) Malpractice.

(C) Off-label testing.

(D) Uncertified testing.

95) An external control determines which of the following?

(A) Whether a test is performed properly.

(B) Whether the electronic functions of the equipment are in working properly.

(C) Whether the sample size is adequate.

(D) All of the above.

96) Which of the following are ways to troubleshoot an incorrect quality-control test?

(A) Recheck compliance with manufacturer instructions.

(B) Visualize the reagent and controls for contamination.

(C) Check the expiration date.

(D) All of the above.

97) Which of the following statements is incorrect regarding waived testing?

(A) Swabs included in the test kits should be used for testing.

(B) Either dermal puncture or venipuncture whole blood is an appropriate sample.

(C) Label the test device (strip or cassette) when it requires directly applying the sample.

(D) A phlebotomist is not authorized to perform a waived test.

98) When is a result considered invalid?

(A) It does not coincide with the patient's clinical presentation.

(B) Quantitative values are beyond the reference range.

(C) Test equipment displays high or low.

(D) All of the above.

99) Which of the following is the next best step when a waived test result is equivocal?

(A) Do not report the results. Repeat the test.

(B) Order a confirmatory test.

(C) Report the results as is.

(D) Perform a quality-control test.

100) Whom among the following performs an external quality assessment?

(A) Colleagues.

(B) A consultant.

(C) Proficiency testing program.

(D) All of the above.

101) You are assigned to collect blood samples for 12 patients in the ward. The patient in bed 8 is unconscious and does not rouse even after a sternal rub. You should do which of the following?

(A) Call for help.

(B) Begin chest compressions.

(C) Check their airway for obstruction.

(D) Check if they are breathing.

102) How deep should chest compressions in children be?

(A) 1.5 inches.

(B) 1.5 cm.

(C) 2 inches.

(D) 2 cm.

103) The rate of chest compressions should be which of the following?

(A) 90 to 100 per minute in adults.

(B) 100 to 120 per minute in children.

(C) 110 to 160 per minute in infants.

(D) All of the above.

104) Which of the following refers to the laboratory's practices designed to guarantee quality patient care?

(A) Quality management.

(B) Quality assessment.

(C) Quality systems essentials.

(D) Quality control.

105) Which of the following organizations develops a set of standards by which every laboratory procedure is measured?

(A) The Joint Commission.

(B) CLSI.

(C) CLIA.

(D) CAP.

106) Which of the following quality assessment procedures compares a patient's old test results with current ones?

(A) Reference range.

(B) Critical values.

(C) Delta check.

(D) Competency assessment.

107) Procedural variables are classified accordingly. Which of the following would a phlebotomist be least involved in?

(A) Pre-examination variables.

(B) Examination variables.

(C) Post-examination variables.

(D) Requisition errors.

108) A description of the principles and purpose for each test can be found in which of the following?

(A) Requisition forms.

(B) Electronic hospital records.

(C) Laboratory report.

(D) Procedural manual.

109) Which of the following documents the laboratory's overall performance?

(A) Quality-management systems.

(B) Quality assessment.

(C) Quality systems essentials.

(D) Quality control.

110) Which of the following systems involved in quality management is designed to decrease costs and eliminate wastes to allow the laboratory to perform better with less and increase customer and staff satisfaction?

(A) Lean system.

(B) Six Sigma.

(C) Root cause analysis.

(D) Nonconforming events.

111) A misidentified patient has a hemolytic transfusion reaction. Which of the following should be the laboratory's next actions?

(A) Fire the phlebotomist who extracted the wrong crossmatch sample.

(B) Fire the nurse who transfused the wrong blood.

(C) Perform a root cause analysis.

(D) Report a nonconforming event.

112) Which of the following is the deepest layer of the skin?

(A) Epidermis.

(B) Dermis.

(C) Subcutaneous layer.

(D) Pericardium.

113) Which of the following conditions refers to an allergic reaction to irritant substances, like soap, cosmetics, or certain plants?

(A) Keloid.

(B) Impetigo.

(C) Eczema.

(D) Dermatitis.

114) Which of the following is the appropriate remedy when a phlebotomist suffers from allergic contact dermatitis to gloves?

(A) They should choose another profession.

(B) They should use a cotton glove liner.

(C) They are exempt from using gloves when performing venipuncture.

(D) They should use powdered gloves.

115) Which of the following conditions refers to a pus-filled skin infection?

(A) Keloid.

(B) Impetigo.

(C) Eczema.

(D) Dermatitis.

116) Which of the following laboratory tests is ordered to determine the extent of muscular damage?

(A) Myoglobin.

(B) Creatinine kinase.

(C) Lactate dehydrogenase.

(D) All of the above.

117) Which of the following components of the peripheral nervous system controls involuntary body functions, such as heart rate, breathing, and digestion?

(A) Autonomic nervous system.

(B) Sympathetic nervous system.

(C) Parasympathetic nervous system.

(D) Afferent nervous system.

118) Which of the following laboratory tests is ordered to measure the body pH in a patient with respiratory failure?

(A) Arterial blood gas.

(B) Bronchoalveolar lavage.

(C) Serum chloride test.

(D) Complete blood count.

119) Which of the following laboratory tests is paired with its correct clinical correlation?

(A) Alkaline phosphatase and multiple myeloma.

(B) Antinuclear antibody and sickle cell disease.

(C) Vitamin D and cystic fibrosis.

(D) Lactate dehydrogenase and CNS disorders.

120) Which of the following laboratory tests is used to estimate the kidneys' function?

(A) Glomerular filtration rate.

(B) Renin.

(C) Erythropoietin.

(D) Creatinine.

Test 2 Answers and Explanations

1) (A) Keeping your workstation neat and organized.

Professional traits of the phlebotomist include being competent and organized. Having a well-organized workspace and tray displays competence. Patients who see you fumbling about for your equipment will have the impression that you are unskilled.

2) (D) Walking tall as they enter a patient's room.

This choice displays positive body language. Remember, you are interacting with a patient for only a few minutes, but the way you walk and carry yourself will leave a message. Walking tall, bearing a warm smile, and maintaining eye contact all display positive body language, which helps patients feel at ease and confident in your skills.

3) (D) All of the above.

Reverse isolation is observed for newborns and patients immunocompromised or receiving chemotherapy. In these areas, all PPE must be sterile. When you are done with phlebotomy, take all your equipment out with you. Remove PPE only after leaving the room. This limits exposure to possible pathogens from outside.

4) (C) Malpractice.

By performing a procedure that the phlebotomist has not been adequately trained to do, they commit an unprofessional act. The patient ends up with a nerve injury, which fulfills the criteria for malpractice, which is the failure to demonstrate skillfulness by a medical professional, resulting in injury or compromise to a patient.

5) (A) A requirement of the laws of your state.

The rules for HIV testing may vary by state, depending on the existing laws. Always keep updated with the HIV consent protocol of your state.

6) (D) Gloves, goggles, gown, mask.

When removing PPE, the most contaminated items must be removed first. Make sure these do not contact your skin. The order for removing is gloves first, then goggles or face shields, gown, and mask.

7) (D) It usually consists of hard hats and reflective gear.

PPE usually consists of a mask, face protection, gown, and gloves. In a medical or chemical setting, PPE also includes a waste bin or a biohazard container. A hard hat and reflective gear are not useful in the laboratory setting.

8) (A) Proper donning of personal protective equipment.

Standard precautions are created on the assumption that every person and surface is contaminated and is a potential source of transmissible infection. Therefore, proper hand hygiene, correct donning of PPE, respiratory hygiene or cough/sneeze etiquette, patient-care apparatus, environmental awareness, and proper handling of textiles and laundry are advised.

9) (A) Mucous membranes around the eyes.

Exposure to blood-borne pathogens should be the highest priority to be wary of while on duty. Blood-borne pathogens may utilize the mucous membranes around the eyes (or lesions on the skin as portals of entry.

10) (A) Clostridium tetani.

In the hospital or laboratory setting, using an alcohol-based hand rub is acceptable when your hands are not visibly dirty. However, alcohol disinfectants are not recommended in case of contact with Clostridium species or spore-forming bacilli such as Clostridium tetani.

11) (C) Wearing artificial nails.

Since you work with your hands throughout the day, you are strongly advised to keep them clean. This can be achieved by having clean and short nails. Wearing artificial nails is not recommended in the hospital setting. These nails and dangling jewelry can be pulled by an irate patient or get tangled with equipment.

12) (D) Airborne precautions.

Airborne precautions are respiratory hazards that can be blocked by employing standard precautions, along with a mask or respirator. Some possible infections that can be prevented with the proper precautions are adenovirus, mumps, chicken pox, tuberculosis, herpes zoster/shingles, and COVID-19.

13) (C) Biological waste.

All equipment contaminated with bodily fluids must be disposed of in containers marked with biohazard symbols. Items such as bandages, used gauze, used PPE, and alcohol pads belong in the biological waste bin. Urine must be disposed of in the sink within the laboratory.

14) (C) Endocrine.

The endocrine system regulates body metabolism, sleep, stress response, and reproductive functions through hormones. The brain (A) is an organ. Red blood is a cell (B), while the epithelium is a type of tissue (D).

15) (D) Transverse.

The human body is described across different planes. The transverse plane is a cross-sectional cut horizontally into upper and lower sections.

16) (D) Femoral.

This artery is located at the inguinal canal and is often used to extract arterial blood.

17) (C) Count the beats again for one full minute.

Normally, the heart rate is measured by counting the number of beats for 30 seconds and then multiplying by 2. However, if the heart rate is irregular, you need to repeat the count for 1 full minute. This is to ensure that the heartbeat's regularity is noted during reporting. Choices A and D are time-consuming and unnecessary. Choice B assumes that the same procedure happens for both regular and irregular heartbeats.

18) (D) 5–6 liters.

This is the average number of liters of blood a human adult usually has. This is the result of blood being composed of plasma, water, and substances like proteins, among others. All other choices are too low for an average adult.

19) (B) D antigen.

The D antigen, or Rh factor, may be present or absent in the erythrocytes. Persons who are Rh-negative do not have naturally occurring antibodies to Rh. They must first encounter Rh-positive blood through transfusion or pregnancy. Afterward, their plasma retains memory in the form of anti-D antibodies, such that a second transfusion of Rh-positive blood results in a transfusion reaction. This may lead to a condition known as a hemolytic disease in the newborn.

20) (A) Alveolar macrophage.

When monocytes are in the tissues, they go by different names. They are alveolar macrophages in the lungs, osteoclasts in the bone, microglia in the CNS, and Kupffer cell in the liver.

21) (C) Fibrin clot.

The cascade ends after factor XIII is activated. At this point, the fibrin clot is stabilized, and the clot retracts or tightens. Evaluation of this stage is possible by measuring the thrombin time.

22) (B) Electrocardiogram.

An electrocardiogram (commonly referred to as an ECG) measures the cardiac cycle. It gives information on the time for one heartbeat, or cardiac cycle, to complete, as well as the regularity of the heart's rhythm. Clinicians determine the timing of each atrial and ventricular systole and diastole by understanding the relationship of the waves and crests on the ECG tracing. An ECG is indispensable for the diagnosis of heart conditions.

23) (A) Pulmonary vein.

The pulmonary vein is the only vein that does not carry deoxygenated blood. It gains the name "vein" because, like all the other veins, it carries blood toward the heart.

24) (A) Short draw.

Expired tubes may have already lost their vacuum, resulting in a short draw. This can interfere with test results.

25) (D) Activate the needle's safety device.

Never recap a needle. Once sample collection is complete, activate the safety device. Dispose of all sharps into designated containers. When using a syringe attached to a transfer device, throw away the whole assembled unit; do not attempt to disassemble it.

26) (C) Pink top.

The pink top contains EDTA and is used as a special label for blood bank tests, such as crossmatching, to avoid the misidentification of patients.

27) (D) Special handling requirements for the tests requested.

The phlebotomist is expected to know and prepare for special handling of certain tests, such as wrapping tubes in foil for photosensitive tests (i.e., bilirubin), sending in an ice slurry, or warming.

28) (D) All of the above.

The most important step is to identify the patient. CLSI standards require two identifiers. Ask every patient to verbally state their first and last names and give their birth date. Compare these to the information written on the patient ID bands and with the requisition forms. You must also obtain permission to proceed with venipuncture.

29) (B) Position the arm so the wrist through the shoulder can be traced with a straight line.

The correct position of the patient's arm should be downward and extended, such that the wrist through the shoulder can be traced with a straight line. This way, your tubes may fill properly and avoid additive carryover. Do not hyperextend their elbows. This may make it difficult to find the veins.

30) (D) All of the above.

You may need to adjust your chosen system. A butterfly system is preferable for very old or very young patients. With patients who have small and thin veins, the syringe system may be a better choice. Also, consider the number of tests needed and the volume of blood to be extracted.

31) (C) Cephalic vein.

The cephalic vein is the second choice for a venipuncture site. It is the most lateral, and it can be difficult to locate. It is also less well-anchored. The basilic vein is the last choice.

32) (A) 60 seconds.

Leaving the tourniquet on too long causes blood cells to hemolyze and results in poor laboratory results. It is recommended that a tourniquet be used only for a maximum of 1 minute.

33) (D) Using the index finger.

After applying the tourniquet, you can find veins on sight or by palpating with your index finger. Veins feel rubbery or spongy and cylindrical. You can feel the vein's direction or orientation and depth. Unlike arteries, veins should not have a pulse. The thumb is not suitable for palpating a vein because the thumb has its own pulse.

34) (A) Wait for 1 minute for the alcohol to dry.

Wait about 1 minute for the alcohol to dry. Do not touch the site, or fan or wipe it. Drying maximizes alcohol's bacteriostatic action. Puncturing a site while the alcohol is still wet (B) causes a stinging sensation, and contamination might cause hemolysis of the specimen.

35) (A) At a 15°- to 30°-angle with the bevel facing up.

To perform the venipuncture, hold the ETS properly and close to the hub. Visualize the needle to be in line with the vein, then insert it smoothly and swiftly, bevel facing up at a 15°- to 30°-angle through the skin into the vein. When it has entered the vein, you can feel the resistance lowering.

36) (A) Immediately after it is removed from the ETS holder.

Invert each tube the appropriate number of times as soon as it has collected blood. These few seconds do not cause any significant discomfort to your patient. It also ensures the integrity of the specimen.

37) (A) 2 hours.

Tubes with anticoagulant additives must be centrifuged within 2 hours. The ideal time for the specimen to reach the laboratory department should be within 45 minutes. This allows time for immediate centrifugation.

38) (D) All of the above.

In the outpatient laboratory, once you have labeled the specimen and bandaged the patient's arm, you may thank the patient for cooperating. Release them with appropriate instructions. Remind them to eat and drink if they had been fasting and have no other procedures to be done for the day. Clean up your work area before the next patient.

39) (D) Verify their information with their photo ID card and see if these match the requisition slip.

In the outpatient setting, patients do not often wear ID bands. Verify their information with proof of identification bearing their photograph in compliance with CLSI standards. This may also be a requirement for legal tests. CLSI standards require two identifiers. Ask every patient to verbally state their first and last names, spell them out, and give their birth date. Compare these to the information written on the patient's ID and with the requisition forms.

40) (A) Wake her gently, identify yourself, and wait for her to be oriented.

When you encounter this situation, you must wake the patient politely. Identify yourself and wait for her to be oriented. You still need to ask her to identify her name and birth date verbally and consent to the procedure. Remember, you can face legal issues for venipuncture without consent. It is important not to skip the patient. Unconscious and expired patients may also appear to be peacefully asleep.

41) (B) Cross-reference their temporary ID number with their permanent number.

In the emergency department, patients may arrive unidentified. The AABB requires each unidentified patient to receive a temporary ID. Some facilities use a temporary name (e.g., John Doe) with a number. After the patient is identified, the facility can issue a unique patient ID number. Take note of the temporary ID on the requisition slip and cross-reference it with the permanent ID number once it becomes available.

42) (B) The patient is well-rested and fasted.

It is preferable to obtain specimens during the basal state. This is when the patient is well-rested and fasted (no food or drinks except water for the last 12 hours). This is often early in the morning. Venipuncture during the basal state achieves the best comparison of patient test values with reference ranges.

43) (D) In crying children, white cell count may be elevated.

This is the only correct statement among the choices.

Choice A: Alcohol intake reduces testosterone.

Choice B: Prolonged fasting causes bilirubin, glucagon, triglycerides, lactate, and ketones to be elevated.

Choice C: Change in position from supine to upright may affect tests that measure protein-bound compounds.

44) (A) Syncope.

Patients often appear pale, hyperventilating, cold, and clammy right before fainting. They may complain of dizziness, blurring or tunnel vision, and nausea. Be wary of these symptoms. Always ensure barriers, such as armrests and bed rails, are used to prevent fall injuries.

45) (A) Probing the needle vigorously.

Hemoconcentration affects many test results. It is caused by probing the needle on the site excessively, venipuncture on sclerotic veins or edematous limbs, and pumping fists.

46) (D) Hand veins.

Do not perform venipuncture in areas with possible infections or contamination or places with low blood flow, such as over hematomas, on edematous limbs, and on sclerosed veins. Small, superficial veins are also found on the dorsum of the hand. These may be a site for venipuncture when no other areas are suitable.

47) (D) Only A and B.

On obese patients, you may need to use a blood pressure cuff or longer bariatric-type tourniquets to locate their veins. Avoid probing. A syringe system with a longer needle may be an alternative.

48) (C) Needle angle too narrow.

When positioning a needle at a very narrow angle, the needle is inserted too close to the skin. You may initially reach the lumen of the vein successfully, but blood will flow too slowly into the collecting tube. This angle allows blood to leak into the tissues. This may create a hematoma.

49) (B) Nerve damage.

Nerve damage is the dreaded complication of venipuncture. You can be alerted to this if the patient complains of tingling, shock-like sensations, or overt pain and numbness. Immediately discontinue venipuncture. Release the tourniquet and remove the tubes and needle.

50) (D) Drawing blood from a sclerosed vein.

The following preventable venipuncture technical errors result in hemolyzed samples:

- Using a 23-gauge needle, which has a too-narrow bore
- Improperly assembled devices
- Pulling a syringe plunger too hard
- Extraction on an area with hematoma
- Shaking evacuated tubes
- Tourniquet used for more than a minute
- Alcohol still wet when venipuncture was performed
- Probing improperly
- Collecting on a sclerosed vein

51) (D) All of the above.

Instances when a dermal puncture is unsuitable include severe dehydration and edematous fingers. A dermal puncture cannot provide adequate blood volume to run tests requiring larger volumes, such as coagulation assays, ESR, and blood cultures.

52) (B) Dermal puncture collects fluid from the tissues as well.

Dermal puncture also collects some interstitial and intercellular fluid (fluids around and within the cells, respectively).

Choice A: Capillary sample analytes require a different set of reference values from venipuncture.

Choice B: Milking the site does not increase blood circulation; instead, it produces a diluted or contaminated sample from introducing tissue fluids.

Choice C: Warming the area, not cooling, before a dermal puncture increases blood circulation.

53) (B) Depth of the puncture.

The depth of puncture should only be a maximum of 2 mm. This avoids reaching the bone and prevents complications of osteomyelitis and osteochondritis. For this reason, phlebotomists should never perform a puncture using uncontrolled surgical blades.

54) (A) Third or fourth finger.

The usual dermal puncture areas are either the heel and the pads of the middle (third) and ring (fourth) fingers. Other fingers are not suitable, since thumbs may be callused, the index fingers contain more nerve endings, and the little fingers contain less tissue. Do not attempt heel punctures on the back of the heel or on the toes and arches, as they are too close to other sensitive structures.

55) (D) All of the above.

The main concern in dermal puncture is avoiding puncturing the bone and consequently introducing a pathogen causing osteomyelitis. Never repeat a puncture on a previous site. This can introduce pathogens and promote infections. A new device must be used for every dermal puncture attempt.

56) (C) It prevents the formation of a round drop of blood.

As with venipuncture, 70% isopropyl alcohol is ideal for cleansing the area. It must be allowed to dry before the procedure. Failing to do so may cause pain, rapid hemolysis, and specimen contamination. This also causes collection difficulties, since the admixture of blood and alcohol prevents the round blood drop from forming.

57) (A) Blood smear, complete blood count, bilirubin.

When drawing capillary blood, blood smears are performed first. A complete blood count sample in lavender EDTA tubes is collected second. Lastly, bilirubin is collected in amber tubes.

58) (A) 24 hours after birth.

Screening for these conditions is performed on a dermal puncture sample taken between 24 and 48 hours after delivery.

59) (C) 30 degrees.

A spreader slide angled at 30 or 40 degrees is used to prepare an adequate peripheral blood smear.

60) (A) To concentrate the sample to find and detect malarial parasites.

Thick smears prepare a concentrated sample to find and detect malarial parasites.

61) (A) Blood culture.

Blood culture results would report the growth or absence of bacteria after every 24 hours. If bacteria were able to grow, further chemical and microscopic analysis would be done to identify the genus and species. Antibiotic susceptibility would also be performed to identify which antibiotic can be used against these bacteria and which antibiotic they can resist.

62) (B) Use sterile yellow (SPS) evacuated tube.

A sterile yellow (SPS) evacuated tube may also be used to collect the sample. This tube contains the same anticoagulant as blood culture bottles—sodium polyanethole sulfonate. The blood is then inoculated onto appropriate culture media in the laboratory. Sodium polyanethol sulfonate is the only suitable anticoagulant for blood cultures because it allows bacterial growth.

63) (B) The aerobic bottle is filled first.

When a winged collection system is used, blood is collected in the aerobic bottle first. This ensures the air present in the tubing does not contaminate the anaerobic bottle.

64) (A) 30 seconds.

A skin cleanser with a mixture of chlorhexidine gluconate and alcohol (ChloraPrep) is available and used to scrub the site using a back-and-forth motion. Allow at least 30 seconds for the cleanser to dry before proceeding.

65) (A) To collect the least amount of blood while maintaining the proper blood-to-culture medium ratio.

Proper volumes must be collected to ensure the correct ratio of blood-to-culture medium is 1:10. This allows bacteria to grow on the culture. Collecting the least amount of blood is important in preventing iatrogenic anemia.

66) (B) Ammonia.

Tests for acetone, arterial blood gases, pyruvate, lactic acid, and ammonia require chilling. For arterial blood gas specimens collected in a plastic syringe and analyzed in 30 minutes, chilling is not required.

67) (A) Porphyrins.

Photosensitive analytes deteriorate upon exposure to light or ultraviolet radiation. These specimens may be wrapped in aluminum foil or collected in amber-colored tubes. Photosensitive analytes include bilirubin, vitamin A, porphyrins, folate, niacin (vitamin B6), and cyanocobalamin (vitamin B12).

68) (A) Paternity testing samples.

Paternity testing samples are commonly collected in yellow (ACD) tubes.

69) (A) They received a vaccine for varicella 2 days ago.

At least 4 weeks should pass after vaccination with live vaccines (MMR, varicella), and at least 2 weeks for live COVID-19 vaccine, rubeola, oral polio vaccine, and yellow fever vaccine before a volunteer can donate blood. If only 2 days have passed, the volunteer should be deferred from donating blood until at least 4 weeks pass.

70) (B) Citrate-phosphate-dextrose.

The blood bag contains citrate-phosphate-dextrose or citrate-phosphate-dextrose-adenine to preserve the blood and prevent clots.

71) (A) Pump their fist to allow hemoconcentration of the blood.

Of the choices, only Option A is correct. The donor is encouraged to pump their fist to allow a faster blood flow. Contrary to venipuncture, hemoconcentration is allowable in blood bank units.

72) (C) Ask the patient to submit a new one.

Urine samples should be submitted to the laboratory within 2 hours. It should be refrigerated if testing cannot be done immediately. This assures the accuracy of the tests. Patients are instructed to submit their urine within 2 hours or refrigerate it if it cannot be delivered within this time.

73) (A) pH of 9.5.

A pH of 9.5 indicates urine tampering. Derangements in urine temperature, color, pH, and specific gravity suggest contamination. Tampering is indicated by urine temperatures of below 32.5°C or above 37.7°C, pH above 9, and specific gravity of <1.005.

74) (D) All of the above.

The patient should refrain from sexual activity for 3 days but not more than 5 days. If the sample is collected at home, instruct the patient to keep it warm (37° C). The sample is collected in a sterile cup.

75) (D) All of the above.

Nasopharyngeal swabs are requested for the detection of respiratory syncytial viruses, influenza viruses, bordetella pertussis, and, more commonly, SARSCOV-2, the virus responsible for COVID-19.

76) (C) Jamshidi needle.

The oncologist or hematologist inserts a thick Jamshidi needle into the iliac crest to take a sample of the patient's bone marrow.

77) (C) Cerebrospinal fluid.

This fluid surrounds the cranial and spinal cord meninges, which serve to cushion these sensitive areas, supply nutrients, and remove metabolic waste. The samples are used to investigate the organisms responsible for meningitis and other neurological pathologies.

78) (B) Tube 2 for microbiology.

CSF is collected in three sterile tubes labeled according to the collection order. The first tube is intended for chemistry and immunoserology assays. The second tube is for microbiology, and the third is for hematology and cytology.

79) (A) Heparin.

Heparin-containing tubes are used for Gram stain and microbiologic culture. Sodium fluoride-containing gray tubes are used for synovial fluid glucose tests. A plain sterile tube is used for other tests.

80) (D) Peritoneal.

An increase in the peritoneal fluid in conditions of hypoproteinemia and lymphatic obstruction is also known as ascites.

81) (A) C-urea breath test.

H. pylori may be detected indirectly through the carbon dioxide content from a breath sample. This test is known as the C-urea breath test.

82) (A) 850 to 1,000 gravity for 10 minutes.

Whole blood from venipuncture may need to be spun for about 10 minutes inside a centrifuge. This machine uses a high centrifugal force (at 850 to 1,000 gravity) to separate the blood cells from the serum or plasma component.

83) (B) Plasma.

Plasma is obtained after centrifugation of blood from anticoagulant-containing tubes.

84) (D) All of the above.

The following are the rules for centrifugation:

- Keep all tubes closed and balance the rotor equally by positioning tubes of equal size and volume across each other.
- Keep the centrifuge covered when operating. This ensures no aerosols or broken glass escapes when a tube breaks inside the machine.
- Observe the centrifuge for any excessive vibration before leaving the area.

85) (C) 48 hours.

Refrigerated serum or plasma should be maintained at 2° C to 8° C if testing is not done after 8 hours. It can be kept for up to 48 hours.

86) (B) 4 hours.

A specimen in EDTA-anticoagulated tubes for CBC may remain at room temperature for up to 24 hours. However, from EDTA microtainers, CBC should be done within 4 hours.

87) (D) Category B is generally not life-threatening.

Biohazardous material may be designated one of two classifications:

Category A. Exposure to these substances may be potentially disabling or life-threatening to humans (UN 2814) or animals.

Category B. Exposure to these substances is not generally disabling or life-threatening to humans or animals.

88) (B) UN 3373 Biological Substance Category B.

Laboratory specimens are biohazardous materials. When shipped in public transport, they should be carried in triple packaging. The third should be a rigid container marked with "UN 3373 Biological Substance Category B."

89) (C) Storing an archive of a patient's health records.

The LIS is a computer application specifically developed for laboratory operations. It can generate laboratory requisitions, prepare labels, and store archives of patient results and health records, among others. While it can make patient ID and communication with health care staff easier, the phlebotomist should perform patient ID and monitor complications by themselves.

90) (C) Moderate complexity.

These procedures require training and understanding of principles and instrument calibration (e.g., automated hematology analyzer, glycohemoglobin analyzer).

91) (B) Glycosylated hemoglobin test.

Moderate complexity procedures require training and understanding of principles and instrument calibration (e.g., automated hematology analyzer, glycohemoglobin analyzer).

92) (A) CLIA.

This stipulates the standards that every laboratory must follow in the course of diagnostic procedures, professional qualifications, quality-management systems, and handling complaints. These are set by the Center for Medicare & Medicaid Services (CMS).

93) (C) To gather data on waived tests.

There are certain circumstances under which CMS will inspect waived testing procedures during its surveillance at dedicated testing sites:

- When a complaint has been raised
- To ascertain whether these sites are performing only the tests they are permitted to (i.e., certified waived tests)
- To gather data on waived tests

94) (C) Off-label testing.

The above situation is an example of off-label testing. This means the FDA did not clear the test kit for this purpose or the manufacturer did not have enough data to support this. Testing capillary blood glucose when the patient's hematocrit levels or oxygen saturation is not within the range described in the manufacturer's instructions may result in unnecessary clinical interventions, which may or may not harm the patient.

95) (A) Whether a test is performed properly.

An external control determines whether a test is performed properly and whether the results fall within the expected range. External controls are provided by the manufacturer and appear like test samples.

96) (D) All of the above.

Troubleshooting often involves:

- Rechecking compliance with the manufacturer's instructions
- Looking at the reagent and controls for contamination
- Rechecking compliance with storage requirements
- Checking expiration date
- Following the manufacturer's troubleshooting instructions

97) (D) A phlebotomist is not authorized to perform a waived test.

After proper training, a phlebotomist may be assigned to perform waived testing.

Choice A: Swabs included in the test kits are not interchangeable with sterile swabs. The differences in the material may provide inaccurate results.

Choice B: Whole blood for waived tests may be collected through dermal puncture or venipuncture

Choice C: For test kits that require direct application of the sample onto the test device (strip or cassette).

98) (D) All of the above.

An invalid result is any of the following:

- A test indicates "invalid."
- It does not coincide with a patient's clinical presentation.
- Quantitative values are beyond the provided range.
- Test equipment displays a high or low result.

Refer to the manufacturer's instructions for this situation. There should be additional steps to perform to arrive at accurate measurements.

99) (B) Order a confirmatory test.

Waived test results may be equivocal. This may mean additional testing or a confirmatory test is required. Your laboratory may have its own policies on when to perform confirmatory tests.

100) (D) All of the above.

An external assessment involves a third party (either a colleague, consultant or a proficiency testing program).

101) (A) Call for help.

If the patient is unresponsive, call for help immediately. This is the priority, as the patient will have a better chance of resuscitation under more experienced hands. Do not leave the patient. Perform the initial survey while waiting for help to arrive.

102) (C) 2 inches.

To perform chest compressions on children, place the heel of either one or two hands (considering the child's size) on the child's lower sternum. Like adult compressions, the depth of compression is 2 inches.

103) (B) 100 to 120 per minute in children.

The rate for chest compressions should be in the range of 100 to 120 per minute. This does not change in children, infants, or adults.

104) (B) Quality assessment.

Quality assessment pertains to the laboratory's practices designed to guarantee quality patient care. It is overseen by The Joint Commission.

105) (B) CLSI.

The Clinical and Laboratory Standards Institute develops a set of standards by which every laboratory procedure is measured. Importantly, if there are any legal proceedings, the regulations outlined in CLSI represent the proper procedures that should have been followed.

106) (C) Delta check.

Delta check compares a patient's old test results with the current results. A variation beyond the established parameter flags the result and alerts personnel to a possible error.

107) (B) Examination variables.

Phlebotomists do not often perform the testing. They are least involved in this aspect unless they are conducting a waived test or point-of-care test.

108) (D) Procedural manual.

This provides a description of the principles and purpose for each test, specimen and collection requirements, a list of materials needed, special precautions (if any), procedure instructions, corrective actions, quality-control methods, and reference ranges.

109) (A) Quality-management systems.

Quality management refers to how a facility adheres to laboratory standards and evaluates the systems to prevent problems and resolve issues. It encompasses quality assessment and quality control.

110) (A) Lean system.

This system involved in quality management is designed to decrease costs and eliminate waste to allow the laboratory to perform better with less and increase customer and staff satisfaction.

111) (C) Perform a root cause analysis.

These events should be reported to The Joint Commission as soon as the event arises and documented for laboratory accreditation purposes. This report provides the following information:

- A description of the sentinel event
- A root cause analysis detailing the actions that could have caused the event
- A detailed action plan

112) (C) Subcutaneous layer.

The skin is composed of three layers. The deepest is the subcutaneous layer. It is made up of fat connecting the organs to the skin. It also functions as a shock absorber, an energy reserve, and insulation.

113) (D) Dermatitis.

Dermatitis, or contact dermatitis, is an allergic reaction to irritant substances, like soap, cosmetics, or certain plants.

114) (B) They should use a cotton glove liner.

A cotton glove liner is available for phlebotomists with allergic dermatitis.

115) (B) Impetigo.

Impetigo is from an infection of *Staphylococcus* or *Streptococcus* bacteria, or both. It presents as a pus-filled lesion that dries to become a yellowish crust.

116) (D) All of the above.

Creatinine kinase, CK-MB, CK-MM, lactate dehydrogenase, and myoglobin are laboratory tests that can determine the extent of muscular damage.

117) (A) Autonomic nervous system.

The autonomic nervous system is a function of the PNS. It controls involuntary body functions, such as heart rate, breathing, and digestion. Its divisions are assigned as sympathetic and parasympathetic.

118) (A) Arterial blood gas.

An analysis of arterial blood gas also generates a measurement of body pH. Adequate respiration ensures the proper levels of gases in the body.

119) (A) Alkaline phosphatase and multiple myeloma.

Only Option A is correct.

120) (D) Creatinine.

Kidney function is estimated through the glomerular filtration rate. This is not a single laboratory test but a value calculated from the patient's weight, age, gender, and creatinine. Creatinine is the correct answer since it is the laboratory test needed to calculate the GFR.

Test 3 Questions

1) Barriers to effective communication include all except which of the following?

(A) Medical jargon.

(B) Hearing loss.

(C) Hand signals.

(D) The patient speaking only Cantonese.

2) A patient does not wish to proceed with blood tests. The phlebotomist should do which of the following?

(A) Ask the orderly to hold the patient down for the procedure.

(B) Document this on the requisition form.

(C) Notify their supervisor immediately.

(D) Ask their colleague to perform the venipuncture.

3) A phlebotomist pretends to be summoned to a celebrity patient's room and simply checks on her while recovering from surgery. The phlebotomist could be accused of which of the following?

A) Defamation.

B) Invasion of privacy.

C) Battery.

D) Negligence.

4) In hand hygiene, alcohol disinfectant is not recommended in case of contact with which bacteria?

(A) *Clostridium tetani.*

(B) *Staphylococcus aureus.*

(C) *Proteus mirabilis.*

(D) *Giardia lamblia.*

5) Which of the following is the proper order for putting on PPE?

(A) Gloves, face shield, mask.

(B) Mask, goggles, gloves.

(C) Face shield, respirator, gown.

(D) Gown, mask, gloves.

6) According to OSHA guidelines, employers must provide free vaccinations for which of the following conditions?

(A) Human papillomavirus.

(B) HIV.

(C) HBV.

(D) HCV.

7) Which of the following precaution categories is employed to avoid infections such as influenza, diphtheria, and scarlet fever?

(A) Emergency precautions.

(B) Standard precautions.

(C) Droplet precautions.

(D) Airborne precautions.

8) Which of the following types of waste refers to parts of the human body that were surgically removed?

(A) Pathologic/anatomical.

(B) Infectious.

(C) Clinical laboratory.

(D) Sharp.

9) The human body is organized so that cells group together to perform more complex functions. This structure is called which of the following?

(A) Tissue.

(B) Muscle.

(C) Organs.

(D) System.

10) The cornea lies superficially on the eyeball. This means which of the following?

(A) The cornea is inside the eyeball.

(B) The cornea is at the midline of the eyeball.

(C) The cornea sits directly on the surface of the eyeball.

(D) The cornea is behind the eyeball.

11) Which of the following planes cuts the body into a right and left section?

(A) Frontal.

(B) Sagittal.

(C) Midsagittal.

(D) Transverse.

12) Which of the following is an artery that goes along the antecubital fossa, with any pulse being felt along the lower edge of the elbow crease?

(A) Radial.

(B) Carotid.

(C) Brachial.

(D) Femoral.

13) When the pulse rate is below 60 bpm in adults, it is referred to as which of the following?

(A) Bradycardia.

(B) Tachycardia.

(C) Arrhythmia.

(D) Bradypnea.

14) Which of the following is the term used when the hemoglobin level in the blood is low?

(A) Leukemia.

(B) Anemia.

(C) Leukocytosis.

(D) Thrombocytosis.

15) Which of the following is a condition that happens when the formation of blood clots obstructs the flow of blood vessels?

(A) Phlebitis.

(B) Thrombosis.

(C) Aneurysm.

(D) Arteriosclerosis.

16) Which of the following blood types is known as the universal donor?

(A) A.

(B) B.

(C) AB.

(D) O.

17) Which of the following white blood cells detoxifies foreign proteins and proliferates in response to allergens and parasites?

(A) Eosinophil.

(B) Lymphocyte.

(C) Monocyte.

(D) Basophil.

18) Which of the following stages of hemostasis is marked by platelet aggregation and the formation of a temporary plug?

(A) Primary.

(B) Secondary.

(C) Fibrin clot.

(D) Clot lysis.

19) When a monocyte is found in the liver tissues, it is often referred to which of the following?

(A) Alveolar macrophage.

(B) Osteoclast.

(C) Microglia.

(D) Kupffer cell.

20) Which of the following tests is used to evaluate the function of the intrinsic coagulation pathway?

(A) Activated partial thromboplastin time.

(B) Prothrombin time.

(C) Thrombin time.

(D) D-dimer.

21) Which of the following tests is used to estimate the extent of fibrinolysis?

(A) Activated partial thromboplastin time.

(B) Prothrombin time.

(C) Thrombin time.

(D) D-dimer.

22) Which of the following statements is correct regarding the difference between arteries and veins?

(A) Veins are larger and thicker.

(B) Arteries are thinner.

(C) The tunica media of arteries contain less elastic tissue.

(D) The veins in the lower limbs contain many valves.

23) Which of the following items are routinely found in a phlebotomist tray?

(A) Flashlight.

(B) Tourniquet.

(C) Urine cups.

(D) Dextrose 50% vials.

24) When asked to collect blood for a metabolic panel in a patient with small veins, the phlebotomist used a 25-gauge needle. Which of the following tests might be affected by this?

(A) Serum potassium and magnesium.

(B) White cell differential counts.

(C) Blood culture and sensitivity.

(D) Crossmatching.

25) Which of the following is the advantage of using the ETS?

(A) The phlebotomist can control the suction pressure manually.

(B) It allows the angle of venipuncture to be lower for difficult veins.

(C) Blood collects directly into the tubes.

(D) Transfer devices allow for the safe transfer of blood.

26) A sample sent to hematology in a lavender top was rejected due to a clot in the tube. Which of the following could be the cause of this?

(A) The phlebotomist failed to invert the tubes eight times.

(B) The phlebotomist used an expired tube.

(C) The phlebotomist had a short draw.

(D) The phlebotomist did not use a discard tube.

27) Which of the following sets of tubes are drawn in the correct order?

(A) Red, orange, yellow, green, light blue, lavender.

(B) Light blue, red, green, lavender, yellow.

(C) Green, lavender, light blue, orange, red, yellow.

(D) Lavender, light blue, green, yellow, orange, red.

28) Which of the following is the first step of venipuncture?

(A) Applying the tourniquet.

(B) Preparing materials.

(C) Greeting the patient.

(D) Obtaining a requisition form.

29) When the patient asks about details of the tests, the phlebotomist should do which of the following?

(A) Describe these using medical jargon to impress the patient.

(B) Tell only the names of the tests to be done.

(C) Politely inform the patient that this information is best given by their physician.

(D) Answer all the patient's questions about their condition.

30) You find out that the patient has not complied with fasting requirements for a blood glucose determination. You should do which of the following?

(A) Reprimand the patient.

(B) Inform the nurse in charge and take the sample.

(C) Take the sample anyway.

(D) Inform the nurse in charge and stand by for further instructions from the physician.

31) Which of the following is the best time to wear your gloves?

(A) In front of the patient.

(B) Before entering a patient's room.

(C) Only before inserting the needle.

(D) Only before handling the blood specimen.

32) Although this vein is superficial and in the antecubital fossa, it is best to be avoided. It is which of the following veins?

(A) Median cubital.

(B) Basilic.

(C) Cephalic.

(D) Axillary.

33) Which of the following happens when the tourniquet is left for longer than one minute?

(A) Hemolysis.

(B) Hemoglobin.

(C) Hematoma.

(D) Skin blanching.

34) Which of the following is the proper orientation of the tourniquet when properly tied around a patient's arm?

(A) The free end is facing away from the antecubital fossa.

(B) The loop touches the antecubital fossa.

(C) The loop is facing upward.

(D) The free end is facing toward the antecubital fossa.

35) To ensure the maximal bacteriostatic action of isopropyl alcohol, it is important to do which of the following?

(A) Wait for 1 minute for the alcohol to dry.

(B) Puncture the site while it is still wet.

(C) Fan the site to dry.

(C) Wipe the site with a cotton pad.

36) Which of the following gives the phlebotomist the idea that the needle has entered the vein?

(A) The resistance on the needle will decrease.

(B) The resistance on the needle will increase.

(C) Blood squirts out of the vein.

(D) A hematoma forms.

37) Which of the following is the appropriate way to apply pressure to the puncture site?

(A) While the needle is in the vein, use gauze and apply pressure for 2 minutes.

(B) Ask the patient to hold down the gauze on the site for about 2 to 3 minutes.

(C) Apply pressure with gauze, then ask the patient to bend their elbow over it.

(D) Keep pressure on the site for 15 seconds.

38) When should each specimen be labeled?

(A) Immediately after each tube is removed from the ETS holder.

(B) On your way to the laboratory.

(C) While you are still with the patient.

(D) In front of the pneumatic tubes.

39) Before leaving an admitted patient, the phlebotomist should do which of the following?

(A) Thank the patient.

(B) Return the bed rails.

(C) Perform hand hygiene.

(D) All of the above.

40) You are asked to do a venipuncture in the psychiatric ward. Which of the following is a prudent practice in this area?

(A) Ask another phlebotomist to accompany you.

(B) Keep your equipment within the patient's reach.

(C) Ask a nurse to help you reassure these patients.

(D) Wait for a family member to give consent to the venipuncture.

41) is it acceptable to have another person verify the identity of which of the following patients?

(A) Teenage patients.

(B) Elderly patients.

(C) 2-month-old patients.

(D) Combative patients.

42) Which of the following is observed when blood is collected too soon after a fatty meal?

(A) Hemolysis.

(B) Lipemia.

(C) Hemoconcentration.

(D) Leukemia.

43) Pre-examination variables affect the integrity of the specimens and alter test results. Which of the following statements is correct?

(A) Reference ranges are the same across age and sex.

(B) Panic attacks may interfere with blood gas levels.

(C) Following short-term exercise, test results are unaffected.

(D) At higher altitudes, oxygen and hemoglobin levels are lower.

44) Your patient appears pale, cold, and clammy as you are about to perform venipuncture. You should do which of the following?

(A) Proceed with the venipuncture.

(B) Instruct the patient to do distracting actions.

(C) Allow them to have a sweet drink.

(D) Instruct the patient to close their eyes.

45) Which of the following tests is affected by prolonged tourniquet application?

(A) Serum cholesterol.

(B) Hemoglobin levels.

(C) Serum potassium.

(D) All of the above.

46) When a patient has IV fluids in both arms, you can which of the following to ensure a proper specimen?

(A) Postpone the venipuncture.

(B) Ask the nurse to hold the IV infusion and draw blood inferior to this point.

(C) Ask the nurse to hold the IV infusion and draw blood above this point.

(D) Use the lower limb veins.

47) Which of the following is a suitable method for cleansing the site for an alcohol level blood test?

(A) Soap and water.

(B) Sodium hypochlorite.

(C) 40% isopropyl alcohol.

(D) Premoistened tissues.

48) Which of the following techniques is recommended when no blood collects into the evacuated tubes after puncturing?

(A) Retry with a tube requiring a larger volume.

(B) Remove the needle immediately and reinsert it.

(C) Probe the needle until there is blood inside the tubes.

(D) Remove the evacuated tube and pull the needle slowly. When it is already just underneath the skin, rotate the needle about a quarter of a turn.

49) Nerve damage is the dreaded complication of venipuncture. Which of the following are some practices you need to avoid?

(A) Probing the needle blindly.

(B) Sudden movements.

(C) Inserting in a lateral direction.

(D) All of the above.

50) Which of the following technical errors leads to a hemolysis formation?

(A) Pulling on a syringe plunger.

(B) Using a 23-gauge needle.

(C) Inverting the evacuated tubes.

(D) Applying alcohol cleanser on the site.

51) On which of the following requested tests would dermal punctures be inappropriate?

(A) ESR.

(B) Blood culture.

(C) Coagulation tests.

(D) All of the above.

52) Which of the following statements is correct?

(A) Newborn blood inherently resists hemolysis.

(B) Capillary blood is a closer representation of a venous sample.

(C) Warming the area before a dermal puncture increases blood circulation.

(D) Milking the site increases blood circulation.

53) All except which of the following equipment is needed for a dermal puncture?

(A) Lancets.

(B) Microtainer® tubes.

(C) Tourniquet.

(D) Alcohol pads.

54) On which sites can a dermal puncture be safely performed on newborns?

(A) Third or fourth fingers.

(B) Earlobes.

(C) The bottom surface of the heel.

(D) Back of the heel.

55) A phlebotomist can prevent infections when performing a dermal puncture by doing which of the following?

(A) Puncturing too deep to hit the bone.

(B) Repeating the puncture on a previous site.

(C) Reusing a lancet.

(D) Waiting for the alcohol to dry before puncturing.

56) For which of the following tests is povidone-iodine recommended for cleansing dermal puncture sites?

(A) Uric acid.

(B) Potassium.

(C) Bilirubin.

(D) All of the above.

57) Which of the following should be the order of draw to collect for blood smear, complete blood count, and capillary blood glucose?

(A) Blood smear, capillary blood glucose, complete blood count.

(B) Capillary blood glucose, blood smear, complete blood count.

(C) Blood smear, complete blood count, capillary blood glucose.

(D) Complete blood count, blood smear, capillary blood glucose.

58) How long must the blood be allowed to air-dry before mailing a newborn screening test?

(A) 15 minutes.

(B) 30 minutes.

(C) 2 hours.

(D) 3 hours.

59) Why does the preparation of blood smears take precedence in the order of draw for dermal punctures?

(A) To avoid collecting blood with platelet clumps.

(B) To avoid carry-over of additives.

(C) To avoid hemolysis.

(D) To ensure the collection of tissue fluid.

60) Which of the following is the use of a thin smear for malarial tests?

(A) To concentrate the sample to find and detect malarial parasites.

(B) To identify the morphology of malarial parasites.

(C) To prevent transmission of blood-borne pathogens.

(D) To use as a medium to grow parasites.

61) The blood culture test results provide the physician with information on which of the following?

(A) Positive growth of bacteria.

(B) Genus and species of bacteria.

(C) Susceptibility or resistance to antibiotics.

(D) All of the above.

62) Which of the following anticoagulants is suitable, as it allows bacteria to grow in blood cultures?

(A) EDTA.

(B) Sodium polyanethol sulfonate.

(C) Acid citrate dextrose.

(D) Sodium fluoride.

63) When it is necessary to take a blood culture sample from patients who are already taking antibiotics, special blood culture bottles are available. These can be which of the following?

(A) An antimicrobial removal device.

(B) Fastidious antimicrobial neutralization.

(C) Polymethylmethacrylate antibiotic beads.

(D) Only A and B.

64) Which of the following are correct practices before collecting specimens for blood culture?

(A) Wipe the rubber stoppers with 70% alcohol after uncapping blood culture bottles.

(B) Wipe the rubber stoppers with iodine after uncapping blood culture bottles.

(C) Do not leave the alcohol pads over these bottles.

(D) It is unnecessary to cleanse the rubber stoppers of the blood culture bottles.

65) Which of the following is the correct blood culture volume requirement for adults?

(A) 8 to 10 mL of blood per blood culture bottle.

(B) 1 mL for every 5 kilograms.

(C) 1 mL for every 10 pounds.

(D) 8 to 10 mL of blood, equally divided into two blood culture bottles.

66) A chilled specimen should not be used for which of the following tests?

(A) ABG.

(B) INR.

(C) ACTH.

(D) PTH.

67) Which of the following tests may require a chain-of-custody form?

(A) Blood alcohol.

(B) Hepatitis panel.

(C) Serum ammonia.

(D) Newborn screening.

68) Which of the following may cause a falsely high blood alcohol level?

(A) Using 70% isopropyl alcohol as a skin cleanser.

(B) Underfilling the gray tube.

(C) Uncapping the tube before testing.

(D) Using Zephiran chloride as a skin cleanser.

69) Which of the following characteristics would make a volunteer eligible to donate blood?

(A) Currently taking warfarin.

(B) Currently taking antibiotics.

(C) Previously donated blood 4 weeks ago.

(D) Currently taking antihypertensive medications.

70) The blood bag should contain which of the following additives to preserve the blood and prevent clots?

(A) Sodium polyanethol sulfonate.

(B) Citrate-phosphate-dextrose-adenine.

(C) Acid citrate dextrose.

(D) Ethylenediaminetetraacetic acid.

71) Which of the following procedures is useful for collecting only platelets from a volunteer?

(A) Apheresis.

(B) Venipuncture.

(C) Electrophoresis.

(D) Centrifugation.

72) A midstream urine specimen is ideal for which of the following tests?

(A) Urine culture.

(B) Drug testing.

(C) Urine pregnancy test.

(D) Routine urinalysis.

73) Which of the following are measures to ensure that urine remains unadulterated for drug testing?

(A) Adding a blueing agent to the toilet reservoir.

(B) Removing water sources from the area.

(C) Ensuring the urine temperature is between 32.5° C and 37.7° C.

(D) All of the above.

74) The patient is instructed to do which of the following for semen collection?

(A) Refrain from sexual activity for 7 days.

(B) Collect the sample in a condom.

(C) Keep the sample warm.

(D) Bring it to the laboratory 2 hours after collection.

75) Which of the following statements regarding semen collection is true?

(A) Taking note of the time of collection is necessary.

(B) The patient should refrain from sexual activity for 7 days.

(C) The sample should be collected only in the laboratory.

(D) Condoms are suitable for semen collection since it is convenient.

76) When assisting with a bone marrow aspiration, which of the following are expected of you?

(A) Prepare 3 or 4 slides for the core biopsy.

(B) Make 6 to 8 thin smears.

(C) Collect 1-2 ml of bone marrow in EDTA and heparin-containing tubes.

(D) All of the above.

77) Amniotic fluid can be used on which of the following tests?

(A) Alpha-fetoprotein.

(B) Bilirubin.

(C) All of the above.

(D) None of the above.

78) Which of the following CSF tubes is correctly paired with its intended department?

(A) Tube 1 for microbiology.

(B) Tube 2 for immunoserology.

(C) Tube 3 for microbiology.

(D) Tube 4 for immunoserology.

79) Synovial fluid should be collected in which of the following tubes to evaluate crystals?

(A) Gray tubes.

(B) Lavender tubes.

(C) Yellow tubes.

(D) Red tubes.

80) Which of the following types of serous fluid is increased by heart failure?

(A) Pleural.

(B) Pericardial.

(C) Parietal.

(D) Peritoneal.

81) The breath can be analyzed for the presence of which of the following conditions?

(A) Alcohol intoxication.

(B) *Helicobacter pylori.*

(C) Lactose intolerance.

(D) All of the above.

82) Which of the following is a less invasive specimen for testing HIV antibodies?

(A) Saliva.

(B) Buccal swab.

(C) Hair.

(D) Dermal puncture.

83) Diagnosis of lactose intolerance from the breath involves which of the following?

(A) An 8-hour fast for a hydrogen breath test.

(B) Hydrogen level being serially measured every 15 minutes for one hour.

(C) Decreasing levels of hydrogen in the balloon, indicating lactose intolerance.

(D) The patient breathing into a balloon device to measure a baseline hydrogen level.

84) Which of the following is obtained after the centrifugation of clotted blood?

(A) Serum.

(B) Plasma.

(C) Buffy coat.

(D) Aliquot.

85) Which of the following statements is true regarding centrifugation?

(A) A clotted tube may be rimmed to allow better separation of serum.

(B) A specimen may be repeatedly centrifuged only two times.

(C) Specimen for whole-blood analysis should not be centrifuged.

(D) Centrifugation may be completed 2 hours after receiving the specimen.

86) How long can serum or plasma be adequately kept at room temperature?

(A) 8 hours.

(B) 24 hours.

(C) 48 hours.

(D) 72 hours.

87) How long can CBC in EDTA tubes remain at room temperature?

(A) 2 hours.

(B) 4 hours.

(C) 8 hours.

(D) 24 hours.

88) How long can glucose count specimens in sodium fluoride tubes be refrigerated?

(A) 12 hours.

(B) 24 hours.

(C) 48 hours.

(D) 72 hours.

89) You should package laboratory specimens to be shipped in public transport in which of the following ways?

(A) In a pneumatic tube capsule.

(B) In a triple packaging.

(C) In a double packaging.

(D) In a biohazard bag.

90) Which of the following functions is the Laboratory Information Systems capable of?

(A) Telling you whether a specimen has already been received in the laboratory.

(B) Viewing the patient's results.

(C) Billing for laboratory services.

(D) All of the above.

91) All except which of the following are waived tests according to CLIA?

(A) COVID-19 rapid antigen test.

(B) Glucometer test.

(C) Urine pregnancy test.

(D) Blood culture.

92) Which of the following is a provider-performed microscopy procedure?

(A) COVID-19 antigen test.

(B) Urine microscopy.

(C) Blood culture and sensitivity.

(D) Complete blood count.

93) Which of the following organizations implements guidelines to prevent infections?

(A) CLIA.

(B) CMS.

(C) OSHA.

(D) CAP.

94) Which of the following are specific rules designed for the conduction of a test kit?

(A) Manufacturer instructions.

(B) Manual of procedures.

(C) Laboratory policies.

(D) All of the above.

95) An internal or procedural control determines which of the following?

(A) Whether a test is performed properly.

(B) Whether the results fall within the expected range.

(C) Whether the sample size is adequate.

(D) All of the above.

96) Quality control ascertains the correctness of test results. Which of the following situations prompts quality-control testing?

(A) When a test shows a result within the range.

(B) After receiving a new shipment of test reagents.

(C) After performing 100 tests of the same lot number.

(D) Every other day.

97) A waived testing can be performed on which of the following samples?

(A) Anticoagulated blood.

(B) Serum.

(C) Nasopharyngeal swabs.

(D) Only A and C.

98) Reading a test kit too early causes an invalid or false negative test because of which of the following?

(A) Test sample and reagent have not completed their chemical reaction.

(B) Colors are underdeveloped or faded.

(C) The reaction moves beyond the visible window.

(D) Colors overdevelop.

99) Which of the following statements is correct?

(A) Qualitative records may be written in symbols ("-" for negative and "+" for positive).

(B) Units may be omitted when recording quantitative values.

(C) Invalid results are recorded along with the results of the repeat test.

(D) Copies of test reports may be shared with anyone who requests them.

100) Which of the following is a notifiable disease?

(A) COVID-19.

(B) Tuberculosis.

(C) Bacillus anthracis.

(D) All of the above.

101) When a patient does not respond to politely waking them up from sleep, the phlebotomist should do which of the following?

(A) Immediately perform a sternal rub.

(B) Immediately give chest compressions.

(C) Immediately shake the patient or try to rouse them with loud noises.

(D) Immediately call the nurse for help.

102) Which of the following is the appropriate time to begin chest compressions?

(A) When a patient does not react to sternal rub.

(B) When a patient is unresponsive and not breathing.

(C) When a patient has a foreign object lodged in their airway.

(D) When a patient has no pulse.

103) The number of rescue breaths if there are multiple responders should be which of the following?

(A) One every 5 seconds.

(B) One every 6 seconds.

(C) Two breaths per 120 compressions.

(D) Two breaths per minute.

104) Which of the following statements regarding cardiopulmonary resuscitation in adults is correct?

(A) Place both hands interlaced on the patient's lower abdomen.

(B) Using the heel of the hand, push on the sternum to depress it at least 2 inches.

(C) The rate should be in a range of 110 to 160 per minute.

(D) All of the above.

105) Which of the following forms the foundations of a quality-management system?

(A) Quality management.

(B) Quality assessment.

(C) Quality systems essentials.

(D) Quality control.

106) The Joint Commission ensures that each laboratory is providing quality care and adhering to which of the following?

(A) National Patient Safety Goals.

(B) Occupational Safety and Health Administration standards.

(C) CLSI standards.

(D) CLIA standards.

107) Which of the following is the most critical error in the laboratory?

(A) Short draw.

(B) Misidentification of a patient.

(C) Mislabeling of specimen.

(D) Improper handling of the specimen.

108) Important components of a laboratory report include all except which of the following?

(A) Patient ID number.

(B) Date and time of collection and results.

(C) Type of specimen.

(D) Name of the nurse in charge of the patient.

109) Errors in identifying a patient whose serum electrolytes are being monitored every 12 hours can be detected by which of the following?

(A) Reference range.

(B) Critical values.

(C) Delta check.

(D) Auto verification.

110) Managing a nonconforming event involves which of the following?

(A) Identifying issues within the laboratory workflow processes.

(B) Implementing changes to these processes and procedures.

(C) Investigating and removing the causes of these nonconforming events.

(D) All of the above.

111) Which of the following tools investigates sentinel events?

(A) Lean system.

(B) Six Sigma.

(C) Root cause analysis.

(D) Nonconforming events.

112) Which of the following pieces of legislation are you violating by showing the patient's diagnosis to her worried son without her consent?

(A) CLIA.

(B) HIPAA.

(C) OSHA.

(D) CAP.

113) How many attempts is the phlebotomist allowed when encountering a difficult venipuncture?

(A) One.

(B) Two.

(C) Three.

(D) Four.

114) Which of the following laboratory tests can detect a complication of renal failure wherein blood contains too much metabolic waste?

(A) Creatinine.

(B) BUN.

(C) Urinalysis.

(D) Electrolytes.

115) Which of the following laboratory tests is paired with its correct clinical correlation?

(A) Creatinine and liver disease.

(B) Cortisol and Cushing's disease.

(C) Pap smear and pregnancy.

(D) TSH and acromegaly.

116) Which of the following conditions causes excruciating abdominal pain and may be due to excessive alcohol intake, gallbladder stones, cancer, or a complication from surgery?

(A) Cholecystitis.

(B) Cholangitis.

(C) Gastroenteritis.

(D) Pancreatitis.

117) Which of the following is a contagious, notifiable, chronic infection due to Mycobacteria causing respiratory problems?

(A) Pulmonary tuberculosis.

(B) Pertussis.

(C) Chronic obstructive pulmonary disease.

(D) Cystic fibrosis.

118) Which of the following hormones produced in the kidneys signals the bone marrows to produce red blood cells?

(A) Renin.

(B) Aldosterone.

(C) Angiotensin.

(D) Erythropoietin.

119) Which of the following bacteria is correctly paired with the sexually transmitted disease it can cause?

(A) *Chlamydia trachomatis* (chlamydia).

(B) *Treponema pallidum* (syphilis).

(C) *Trichomonas vaginalis* (trichomoniasis).

(D) All of the above.

120) Which of the following forms most of the blood and is mostly water with some dissolved substances?

(A) Plasma.

(B) White blood cells.

(C) Hemoglobin.

(D) Erythrocytes.

Test 3 Answers and Explanations

1) (C) Hand signals.

Common barriers include age and educational achievement, hearing loss (B), language, and emotions that may affect verbal communication.

These may be overcome by:

- Avoiding the use of medical jargon
- When speaking to children, try to use age-appropriate lines
- Speaking clearly and looking at the patient while speaking
- Writing down in big print or using hand signals for patients who are hard of hearing
- Asking for the assistance of an interpreter for patients who cannot speak English
- Speaking calmly and reassuring the anxious patient

2) (B) Document this on the requisition form.

When a patient refuses to have blood extracted even after you have explained it, you cannot force it. Having the orderly hold the patient down is inhumane, and you could be sued for battery and assault (A). Instead, you must accept the patient's wishes, inform the nurse and document the patient's refusal. Notifying your supervisor (C) and asking your colleague to perform the venipuncture (D) is unnecessary, as it is the patient's right to refuse.

3) (B) Invasion of privacy.

Under the Tort Law, a patient has the right to be hidden from public exposure. By unrightfully pretending to be part of the patient's healthcare team, the phlebotomist can be charged with invading privacy.

4) (A) *Clostridium tetani.*

In the hospital or laboratory setting, using an alcohol-based hand rub is acceptable when your hands are not visibly dirty. However, alcohol disinfectants are not recommended for contact with *Clostridium* species or spore-forming bacilli, such as *Clostridium tetani.*

5) (D) Gown, mask, gloves.

When putting on PPE, take note of the following steps in proper order:

- Gown
- Mask
- Respirators, goggles, and face shields, if needed
- Gloves

6) (C) HBV.

A vaccine is available for HBV. It is provided free of charge to exposed employees, as mandated by OSHA.

7) (C) Droplet precautions.

Droplets, like airborne infections, enter your skin, eyes, or nose after you touch secretions from infected individuals. Standard precautions are crucial, along with a mask or respirator. Ensure hand hygiene. Possible infections from droplets include adenovirus, mumps, chicken pox, tuberculosis, herpes zoster/shingles, and COVID-19.

8) (A) Pathologic/anatomical.

Pathologic or anatomical waste refers to parts of the human body that have been surgically or accidentally removed, such as tissues, tumors, organs, or placenta.

9) (A) Tissue.

Oftentimes, similar cells group together to perform more complex functions. In this case, they are called tissues.

10) (C) The cornea sits directly on the surface of the eyeball.

The directional term *superficial* was used, which describes something on the surface. Therefore, the cornea sits directly on the surface of the eyeball.

11) (B) Sagittal.

The human body is described across different planes. Imagine there is a flat surface according to different parts of the body and organs. The sagittal plane cuts the body into right and left sections.

12) (C) Brachial.

To determine blood pressure, this artery may be compressed by a blood pressure cuff or sphygmomanometer. The radial artery (A) is an artery that runs along the lateral side of the wrist. The carotid artery (B) is an artery branching near the aorta, while the femoral artery (D) is located at the inguinal canal.

13) (A) Bradycardia.

Bradycardia refers to a pulse rate below 60 bpm, while tachycardia is a rate above 100 bpm. Arrhythmia is the clinical term when the heart is beating with an irregular rhythm. Bradypnea is the clinical term for decreased respiratory rate.

14) (B) Anemia.

This is the term used when the hemoglobin levels are low.

Option A is a type of cancer resulting from a dysregulated increase of leukocytes

Option C refers to leukocytes increasing in response to infections

Option D refers to an increase in platelets.

15) (B) Thrombosis.

This refers to blood clots obstructing the flow of blood through the vessels

Option A: Phlebitis, pain and swelling of the vein can also be caused by an indwelling IV cannula.

Option C: Aneurysm is an outpouching of a blood vessel wall layer due to weakness.

Option D: Arteriosclerosis refers to a hardened, or sclerotic, artery wall.

16 (D) O.

Blood type O is known as the universal donor blood type because it contains no antigens. It cannot form a transfusion reaction with the receiver's plasma.

17) (A) Eosinophil.

Eosinophils form only 1% to 3%, but they have unique responsibilities. They detoxify foreign proteins and proliferate in response to allergens and parasites.

18) (A) Primary.

The primary stage of hemostasis occurs immediately after an injury. The vasculature constricts to prevent blood from leaking out from the injured area. Platelets aggregate and clump together (aggregation). They adhere to the injured area (adhesion) as a temporary plug.

19) (D) Kupffer cell.

When monocytes are in the tissues, they go by different names. They are alveolar macrophages in the lungs, osteoclasts in the bone, microglia in the CNS, and Kupffer cell in the liver.

20) (A) Activated partial thromboplastin time.

The activated partial thromboplastin time (APTT) can estimate the function of the intrinsic pathway. The prothrombin time can estimate the function of the extrinsic pathway and is useful in monitoring the response to warfarin therapy.

21) (D) D-dimer.

Once the blood vessel has healed from the initial insult, the fibrin clot is broken down into fibrin degradation products during fibrinolysis. Therefore, measurement of fibrin degradation products and its protein fragment, D-dimer, can provide an estimate of the extent of fibrinolysis.

22) (D) The veins in the lower limbs contain many valves.

Only Option D is correct. The arteries are larger and thicker blood vessels. The tunica media is more muscular and elastic. The veins are thinner, with tunica media containing less elastic tissue as it is not subjected to higher pressure.

23) (B) Tourniquet .

Routine equipment for venipuncture includes evacuated tube holders, needles, and evacuated tubes for collection using the ETS, different-sized syringes, butterfly set, tourniquets, antiseptic skin preparation solutions, gloves, gauze pads, slides, markers, transfer devices, and a sharps disposal container. The phlebotomist is not expected to carry flashlights (A), urine collection cups (C), or vials of dextrose 50% (D).

24) (A) Serum potassium and magnesium.

The use of 25-gauge needles is generally avoided, as the narrow diameter may cause hemolysis. This may affect the results of serum electrolytes, which leak out from the hemolyzed red blood cells and result in falsely elevated potassium and magnesium. It also causes a false decrease in red cell count, hematocrit, and APTT values.

25) (C) Blood collects directly into the tubes.

The most common venipuncture method is the evacuated tube system. This system relies on a predetermined vacuum that automatically fills each evacuated tube. It does not allow the phlebotomist to control the suction pressure manually (A). The winged collection set allows the angle of venipuncture to be lower for difficult veins (B). The ETS eliminates manual specimen transfer, thereby decreasing the risk of exposure to biological hazards. It does not need a transfer device (D).

26) (A) The phlebotomist failed to invert the tubes eight times.

Anticoagulants prevent the formation of a blood clot by binding calcium (ethylenediaminetetraacetic acid) or inhibiting thrombin (heparin). Tubes containing anticoagulants must be inverted appropriately to mix and prevent microclots. Do not shake. Shaking may cause hemolysis. The formation of air bubbles through the tube while inverting ensures adequate mixing. These tubes must be immediately inverted properly to mix the sample. Lavender tops need to be inverted eight times to prevent microclots. Using expired tubes results in a short draw. An underfilled lavender tube results in the shrinkage of erythrocytes, which can cause false counts. This does not cause clots.

27) (B) Light blue, red, green, lavender, yellow.

The standard order of draw is as follows:

- Sterile blood culture tubes or yellow (SPS)
- Light-blue top
- Serum tubes with or without gel; red/gray, gold, red (plastic), red (glass), orange rapid serum tube, royal blue (clot activator)
- Green, light green, royal blue (heparin)
- Lavender, pink, royal blue (EDTA), tan

- Gray
- Yellow

28) (D) Obtaining a requisition form.

Venipuncture begins when a phlebotomist receives the requisition form. This form outlines the tests to be done as requested by a physician. All the other choices are necessary, but step one should be receiving the requisition form.

29) (C) Politely inform the patient that this information is best given by their physician.

If questioned about which tests are requested and the reasons, politely inform the patient that this information is best given by their physician. Patients can often look up the names of the tests on the internet, which often causes unnecessary anxiety.

30) (D) Inform the nurse in charge and stand by for further instructions from the physician.

Verify special preparations. These include appropriate fasting and skipping medications. In cases when the patient has not complied, report it to the nurse. If the nurse informs you that the physician still requires the specimen, document it on the requisition form and the specimen label as "not fasting."

31) (A) In front of the patient.

Perform hand hygiene in front of the patient, then apply a pair of gloves. Wearing gloves and changing these between patients is a mandate from OSHA. Pull these over your lab coat or protective gown's cuffs. It minimizes any areas of contact with your bare skin.

32) (B) Basilic.

The basilic is the least well-anchored of the three choice veins. It tends to be moveable and may roll away when a needle is inserted, which contributes to a hematoma. It is nearer the nerves and the brachial artery. This site causes the most complications and complaints than the other veins listed.

33) (A) Hemolysis.

Leaving the tourniquet on too long causes blood cells to hemolyze and results in poor laboratory results. It is recommended that a tourniquet be used for a maximum of 1 minute, or 60 seconds. Following this principle, you first use the tourniquet to choose your venipuncture site. Then you reapply it right before you draw blood. CLSI recommends waiting for at least 2 minutes, or 120 seconds, before reapplying the tourniquet.

34) (A) The free end is facing away from the antecubital fossa.

To properly apply the tourniquet, place it flat around the patient's arm, ensuring it is centered. Grasp both ends and pull to create tension. Tuck one side under the other to form a downward-facing loop. This makes sure that the free end is away from the antecubital fossa.

35) (A) Wait for one minute for the alcohol to dry.

Drying maximizes alcohol's bacteriostatic action. Puncturing a site while the alcohol is still wet causes a stinging sensation, and contamination might cause hemolysis of the specimen.

36) (A) The resistance on the needle will decrease.

To perform the venipuncture, hold the ETS properly close to the hub. Position the needle in line with the vein. The needle bevel should be facing upward at a 15°- to 30°-angle. Insert the needle smoothly and swiftly through the skin with one motion. When it has entered the vein, you can feel the resistance lowering.

37) (B) Ask the patient to hold down the gauze on the site for about 2 to 3 minutes.

Ensure the needle is removed from the vein before applying any pressure to the site. Keep pressure on the site; or, if the patient is capable, ask them to hold down the gauze for about 2 to 3 minutes. Bending the elbow is not advisable. It does not provide enough pressure to prevent blood from leaking into the tissues. This causes a hematoma.

38) (C) While you are still with the patient.

You must label each tube right after collecting the specimen and before leaving the patient. Carefully compare your labels with the patient's ID band. You may show your labels to the patient and verbally ask for confirmation as an additional identifying step.

39) (D) All of the above.

When you are finished with the venipuncture, collect all used supplies and discard them in the appropriate containers. Remove your gloves and discard them as well. Perform hand hygiene. Return the bed rails if you have lowered them to make sure the patient does not fall. Forgetting to do this may subject you to legal issues. Thank the patient as you leave their room.

40) (C) Ask a nurse to help you reassure these patients.

In psychiatric wards, it is better to ask a nurse (not your fellow phlebotomist) to help you reassure these patients. The patients are usually anxious and would be reassured by the presence of a familiar person, such as the nurse. Remember to keep your equipment, especially sharps, far from these patients' reach.

41) (C) 2-month-old patients.

For patients who are too young to speak, have cognitive impairments, or cannot speak English, CLSI requires patient information to be provided by a caregiver. In some instances, the nurse may verify the patient's identity. You must document the informant's name on the requisition form.

42) (B) Lipemia.

When blood is collected too soon after a meal (especially one with fried, greasy food and dairy), it may appear cloudy. This is termed lipemia, referring to the high lipid content of the blood sample. This interferes with test results.

43) (B) Panic attacks may interfere with blood gas levels.

Panic attacks may result in hyperventilation and interfere with arterial blood gas results. Consequently, lactate and fatty acids are elevated.

Option A: Reference ranges are varied for each subset of patients. Age and sex affect laboratory tests due to differences in fluid composition, hormones, and body mass.

Option C: Exercise affects laboratory values depending on the extent of vigorous activity, the patient's body type and muscle mass, and the timing of blood collection.

Option D: At higher altitudes, oxygen levels are lower, but hemoglobin and hematocrit counts are higher.

44) (B) Instruct the patient to do distracting actions.

Syncope is a common situation during venipuncture. When your patient shows the symptoms of fainting before the procedure, instruct them to breathe deeply, clench and unclench their thighs, turn their ankles gently clockwise and counterclockwise, or do other distracting actions for comfort. For those outpatients who have fasted and feel faint, let them have a sweet drink after you have succeeded in collecting blood. Ask them to stay in the facility for observation for about 15 to 30 minutes.

45) (D) All of the above.

A prolonged tourniquet causes hemolysis, which leaks potassium, lactate, and certain enzymes out from the cell. After 1 minute, hemoglobin increases by 3%; after 3 minutes, it increases by 7%. Leaving the tourniquet for 2 minutes elevates cholesterol by up to 5% and as high as 15% after only 5 minutes.

46) (B) Ask the nurse to hold the IV infusion and draw blood inferior to this point.

When necessary, you may draw blood inferior to the IV infusion point and, if possible, in another vein. CLSI standards state that you should ask the nurse to interrupt the IV infusion for about 2 minutes before the venipuncture. Document the situation on the requisition form as "specimen collected below the IV infusion point."

47) (A) Soap and water.

Do not use isopropyl alcohol to cleanse the skin for venipuncture to collect blood for alcohol levels. This can potentially interfere with the results. For this test, cleansing with soap and water is preferred. Some laboratories utilize benzalkonium chloride or povidone-iodine as cleansers.

48) (D) Remove the evacuated tube and pull the needle slowly. When it is already just underneath the skin, rotate the needle about a quarter of a turn.

You may easily remedy a wrong angle or a downward-facing bevel by removing the evacuated tube and pulling the needle slowly. When it is already just underneath the skin, redirect your needle or rotate the needle about a quarter of a turn. This fixes the needle position and allows you to adjust your angle so that blood may flow into the tubes. When you suspect the vein has collapsed, retry the collection with a tube requiring lesser volume.

49) (D) All of the above.

Nerve damage is preventable by following the proper venipuncture techniques. Always avoid probing blindly or vigorously, inserting in a lateral direction, and making sudden movements. But when encountered, apply a cold compress to the site. Instruct the patient or request the nurse to use a warm compress after a few hours. Report the incident to the nurse for medical attention and properly document it per your facility's protocols.

50) (B) Using a 23-gauge needle.

Preventable errors resulting in hemolyzed samples:

1. Using a 23-gauge needle, which has a too-narrow bore
2. Improperly assembled devices
3. Pulling a syringe plunger too hard
4. Extraction on an area with hematoma
5. Shaking evacuated tubes
6. Tourniquet used for more than a minute
7. Alcohol still wet when venipuncture was performed
8. Probing improperly
9. Collecting on a sclerosed vein

51) (D) All of the above.

A dermal puncture cannot provide adequate blood volume to run tests requiring larger volumes (coagulation assays, ESR, blood culture).

52) (C) Warming the area before a dermal puncture increases blood circulation.

Warming the area before a dermal puncture increases blood circulation; this produces a better representative sample.

The other options are wrong.

Option A: Newborn blood is inherently fragile and more prone to hemolysis.

Option B: Capillary blood is a closer representation of an arterial sample, not a venous one.

Option D: Milking produces a diluted sample by introducing tissue fluids.

53) (C) Tourniquet.

A tourniquet is not necessary for the dermal puncture procedure.

54) (C) The bottom surface of the heel.

The heel is ideal for dermal puncture in infants because it provides more space between the skin and bone than the fingers. Do not attempt heel punctures on the back of the heel, as it is too close to other sensitive structures. Earlobe punctures are not recommended.

55) (D) Waiting for the alcohol to dry before puncturing.

Drying maximizes alcohol's bacteriostatic action, thereby decreasing the risk of infections. All other options increase the risk of infections in patients by introducing pathogens.

56) (D) All of the above.

Povidone-iodine is not recommended in dermal punctures. It causes altered test results for uric acid, bilirubin, phosphorus, and potassium.

57) (B) Capillary blood glucose, blood smear, complete blood count.

The order of draw for capillary blood is as follows:

- Capillary blood glucose
- Blood smear
- Lavender
- Heparinized tubes (green, mint green, or amber with mint-green cap)
- Gray
- Serum tubes (gold or amber with gold cap)
- Red

Capillary blood glucose is performed before the blood smears. A complete blood count may be collected in a lavender EDTA tube.

58) (D) 3 hours.

After filling all the circles, air-dry the card horizontally. Shield it from direct sunlight. After at least 3 hours, you may seal it in its designated mailing envelope to be sent to the testing laboratory.

59) (A) To avoid collecting blood with platelet clumps.

From dermal punctures, collecting the blood smear sample takes priority over any other tubes. This is to avoid platelet clumps.

60) (B) To identify the morphology of malarial parasites.

Thin smears are used to identify malarial parasites based on their morphologic characteristics.

61) (D) All of the above.

Blood culture results would report the growth or absence of bacteria after every 24 hours. If bacteria were able to grow, further chemical and microscopic analysis would be done to identify the genus and species. Antibiotic susceptibility would also be performed to identify which antibiotic can be used against these bacteria and which antibiotic they can resist.

62) (B) Sodium polyanethole sulfonate.

Sodium polyanethole sulfonate is the only suitable anticoagulant for blood cultures because it allows bacterial growth. Other anticoagulants, like ACD, EDTA, and sodium fluoride, are not suitable because they may inhibit the growth of bacteria.

63) (D) Only A and B.

Special blood culture bottles are available when it is necessary to take a blood culture sample from patients who are already taking antibiotics. These may contain resins (antimicrobial removal devices) or activated charcoal (fastidious antimicrobial neutralization) that are designed to inactivate antibiotics.

64) (A) Wipe the rubber stoppers with 70% alcohol after uncapping blood culture bottles.

When preparing equipment, the rubber stoppers of each blood culture bottle must also be cleansed with 70% alcohol after removing the plastic caps. Do not use iodine to cleanse the rubber stoppers. It can contaminate the specimen or deteriorate the rubber.

Leave the alcohol pad to cover these bottles while you perform the venipuncture. Remove the pad only when you are ready to inoculate the specimen into the bottles.

65) (A) 8 to 10 mL of blood per blood culture bottle.

In adults, 8 to 10 mL of blood is collected per blood culture bottle.

66) (B) INR.

Factor VII may be activated in lower temperatures. Chilling is not recommended for testing prothrombin time and INR.

67) (A) Blood alcohol.

You may be asked to collect forensic samples for use in legal proceedings. These are often tests for blood levels of drugs and alcohol or DNA samples. Follow the policies with extreme care. Specimen handling is documented extensively on the chain-of-custody form.

68) (A) Using 70% isopropyl alcohol as a skin cleanser.

When collecting samples for blood alcohol levels, the site is cleansed with solutions other than 70% isopropyl alcohol. This may be soap and water or benzalkonium (Zephiran) chloride. Zephiran chloride is the recommended skin cleanser and will not affect the test results. Underfilling and uncapping the tubes allow alcohol to escape into the surrounding air, resulting in falsely low blood alcohol levels.

69) (D) Currently taking antihypertensive medications.
Volunteers may continue taking antihypertensive medications, provided their blood pressure falls within the eligible range of at least 90/50 but below 180/100 mmHg.

Option A: Volunteers with bleeding conditions or who take blood thinners, such as warfarin, are not allowed to donate. But a donation of whole blood is allowable while on aspirin.

Option B: Volunteers taking antibiotics for infections must wait until they have taken the last pill of a full course before being eligible.

Option C: Four weeks is not enough time for a person's stores of blood cells to be replenished. At least 8 weeks should pass after a volunteer's last blood donation.

70) (B) citrate-phosphate-dextrose-adenine.

The blood bag contains citrate-phosphate-dextrose or citrate-phosphate-dextrose-adenine to preserve the blood and prevent clots. Sodium polyanethole sulfonate (B) provides anticoagulation for microbiology cultures because it inhibits the destruction of microbes. This will allow bacteria growth, which is not ideal in blood bags. Acid citrate dextrose (C) is found in yellow evacuated tubes, which provides anticoagulation by binding calcium while stabilizing erythrocytes. It is not enough to store blood in the blood bags for extended periods. Ethylenediaminetetraacetic acid (D) is found in lavender evacuated tubes, preventing blood clots for hematology tests.

71) (A) Apheresis.

Of the choices, only (A) is correct. Apheresis is a method of collection for only a specified blood component. It may be collecting units with purely red cells, platelets, or plasma. While centrifugation allows the separation of plasma and serum from the blood, it cannot separate the platelets from the plasma.

72) (A) Urine culture.

A clean-catch midstream sample is ideal for urine cultures since it avoids contamination from external genitalia and the first and last parts of the urinary stream, which may collect surrounding organisms and cells.

73) (D) All of the above.

To ensure that no specimen tampering can happen, drug testing toilets have a blueing agent added to the reservoir. There should be no available water source in the area. The patient is asked to give the sample immediately. Within 4 minutes, the temperature of the sample is checked. If it is below 32.5° C or above 37.7° C, the collector is alerted to possible contamination.

74) (C) Keep the sample warm.

If the sample was collected at home, the patient is instructed to keep it warm (37° C) and bring it to the laboratory within the hour, not after 2 hours. The patient should refrain from sexual activity for 3 days but not more than 5 days. Condoms are not suitable, since they may contain spermicides.

75) (A) Taking note of the time of collection is necessary.

Instruct the patient to take note of the time of collection. When you receive the sample, record both the time of sample collection and the time it arrived. The lifespan of spermatozoa and liquefaction time are time-bound parameters of semen analysis.

76) (D) All of the above.

Your tasks during bone marrow aspiration include:

- Preparation of 3 or 4 slides for the core biopsy
- Preparation of thin smears
- Collection of 1-2 ml of bone marrow in EDTA and heparin-containing tubes

77) (C) All of the above

From the amniotic fluid, alpha-fetoprotein levels and bilirubin levels are quantified to investigate fetal development.

78) (C) Tube 3 for microbiology.

When a fourth tube is collected, the tubes are labeled differently. The first and last tubes are sent to hematology. This allows a comparison to determine contamination with red cells, especially after a traumatic collection. The second tube is for chemistry and immunoserology, while the third tube is for microbiology.

79) (B) Lavender tubes.

Either EDTA- or heparin-containing tubes are used for cell count and identification of crystals from synovial fluid.

80) (B) Pericardial.

Pericardial effusion is the increase in pericardial fluid during disease states, such as heart failure and pericarditis.

81) (D) All of the above.

H. pylori may be detected indirectly through the carbon dioxide content from a breath sample. Increasing levels of hydrogen indicate malabsorption or indigestion of lactose in the gastrointestinal tract. This may aid in diagnosing lactose intolerance, small intestine bacterial overgrowth, and dumping syndromes. Alcohol may be detected in breath-collecting devices often carried by law enforcers.

82) (A) Saliva.

Salivary samples are a less invasive test for the detection of HIV antibodies.

83) (D) The patient breathing into a balloon device to measure a baseline hydrogen level

The hydrogen breath test requires a 12-hour fasting period, not 8.

The procedure is as follows:

1. The patient breathes into a balloon device to measure a baseline hydrogen level
2. The patient ingests lactose
3. The patient breathes into the balloon device, and the hydrogen level is serially measured every 15 minutes over 3 to 5 hours

Increasing levels, not decreasing, indicate malabsorption or indigestion of lactose.

84) (A) Serum.

Serum is obtained after centrifugation of clotted blood.

85) (C) Specimen for whole-blood analysis should not be centrifuged.

Only Option C is true.

Option A: A clotted tube should not be rimmed. This can lead to hemolysis.

Option B: A specimen should not be repeatedly centrifuged. This can alter the test results.

Option D: Centrifugation must be completed within, not after, 2 hours of receiving the specimen to avoid changes in analytes.

86) (A) 8 hours.

Serum or plasma can be kept at room temperature (27° C) for up to 8 hours.

87) (D) 24 hours.

Specimens in EDTA-anticoagulated tubes for CBC may remain at room temperature for up to 24 hours. Note that for some tubes, a CBC should be done within 6 hours.

88) (C) 48 hours.

Specimens in sodium fluoride tubes for glucose determinations may remain at room temperature for up to 24 hours. Refrigeration may extend this limit up to 48 hours.

89) (B) In a triple packaging.

Laboratory specimens are biohazardous materials. The DOT strictly regulates their packaging and labeling. When shipped in public transport, they should be carried in triple packaging. The primary packaging should be leak-proof and have a secure closure, such as tubes or screw-top cups. It should be enclosed in a second leak-proof container, such as a biohazard bag. The third should be a rigid container marked with "UN 3373 Biological Substance Category B."

90) (D) All of the above.

The LIS is a computer application developed explicitly for a laboratory's operation. This application is capable of the following:

- Generating laboratory requisitions
- Preparing labels to be printed out
- Monitoring the current status of a specimen, whether received, being processed, or completed
- Interfacing with automated analyzers with which results are directly reported or verified
- Generating reports
- Storing an archive of a patient's health records
- Preparing bills for services
- Viewing results
- Monitoring compliance with quality-control procedures

91) (D) Blood culture.

Waived testing includes simple diagnostic procedures where little to no training is required. There is little to no risk of error when following the box instructions. Examples include COVID-19 rapid antigen test, home pregnancy test, and glucometer testing. A blood culture is an example of a high-complexity test. Its procedure utilizes complex instrumentation. Interpretation requires higher levels of understanding. The performance of these tests is subjected to proficiency testing. An example is blood culture and antibiotic sensitivity testing.

92) (B) Urine microscopy.

Provider-performed microscopy procedures require the use of a microscope and are performed by a physician or a dentist in their office. An example is urine microscopy.

93) (C) OSHA.

OSHA has implemented guidelines to prevent infections and reduce disease transmission.

94) (A) Manufacturer instructions.

Manufacturer instructions are specific rules recommended by the manufacturer for a test kit. These vary among different manufacturers, even for the same tests. These may even vary for different lots or shipments of a test kit from the same manufacturer.

95) (C) Whether the sample size is adequate.

An internal or procedural control determines whether a test is working properly, the sample size is adequate, and, when applicable, the electronic functions of the equipment are in proper working condition.

96) (B) After receiving a new shipment of test reagents.

Quality-control testing is scheduled regularly with consideration of the following:

- Manufacturer instructions
- When checking the validity of the test
- After environmental changes (such as electrical outages and refrigerator issues)
- For every trainee or new personnel who will be performing the test
- With every shipment of test kits or test reagents

97) (D) Only A and C.

Waived tests should be done only on unprocessed samples, such as:

- Whole blood
- Anticoagulated blood
- Urine
- Feces
- Swabs either from the throat, nasopharynx
- Saliva
- Gastric tissue biopsy

98) (A) Test sample and reagent have not completed their chemical reaction.

Reading a result before the indicated time results in an invalid or false negative test. There has not been enough time for the sample and reagent to complete their chemical reaction.

99) (D) Copies of test reports may be shared with anyone who requests it.

Recording results should be as follows:

- Quantitative values are recorded in standardized units.
- Qualitative results are recorded with words or letters rather than symbols (e.g., "Pos" to indicate positivity or "NR" to indicate "nonreactive").
- Invalid results are recorded as well, along with the results of the repeat test, but report only the correct result.

100) (D) All of the above.

Public health agencies have flagged certain diseases as notifiable. Testing sites are required to report confirmed positive or reactive results for infectious diseases, such as COVID-19, tuberculosis, active viral hepatitis, anthrax, and botulism, among others. Keep updated with your local public health agency for the current list of notifiable diseases.

101) (C) Immediately shake the patient or try to rouse them with loud noises.

When you encounter a sleeping patient, you should wake them up politely. Unconscious and expired patients may also appear to be peacefully asleep. If it is difficult to rouse a patient, try making a loud noise, shaking them, or pinching their earlobe. If they do not respond, elicit pain by performing a sternal rub.

102) (B) When a patient is unresponsive and not breathing.

If the patient is unresponsive and not breathing, immediately being chest compressions.

103) (B) One every 6 seconds.

In the hospital, there will be staff available to take over after this point. It is important to learn the steps, as you may be needed to assist throughout.

104) (B) Using the heel of the hand, push on the sternum to depress it at least 2 inches.

To perform chest compressions, place both hands interlaced on the patient's lower sternum. Using the heel of one hand, push on the sternum to depress it at least 2 inches. Allow the chest to recoil fully. This manually pumps the heart to allow blood to circulate. The rate should be in the range of 100 to 120 per minute.

105) (C) Quality systems essentials.

This forms the foundations of a quality-management system. This involves the interplay of the 12 aspects.

106) (A) National Patient Safety Goals.

Every two years, a survey team from The Joint Commission visits the laboratories to assess their adherence to the National Patient Safety Goals and renew their accreditation.

107) (B) Misidentification of a patient.

Patient misidentification is the most serious error in the laboratory setting.

108) (D) Name of the nurse in charge of the patient.

A laboratory report must include the following information

- Patient identifiers (full name, date of birth)
- Patient ID number
- Date and time of collection

- Date and time of results
- Type of specimen
- If a specimen was rejected, its condition
- Name of test performed
- Results of test
- Reference range or normal values

It does not include the name of the nurse in charge of the patient.

109) (C) Delta check

Delta check compares a patient's old test results with the current results. A variation beyond the established parameter flags the result and alerts personnel to a possible error.

110) (D) All of the above.

In compliance with quality-management systems, laboratories are required to develop a program to manage non-conforming events. This involves identifying issues within the laboratory workflow processes and improving these to provide better patient care and ensure the safety of patients and staff. It also includes the implementation of changes to these processes and procedures. Finally, it serves to investigate and remove the causes of these nonconforming events.

111) (C) Root cause analysis.

Root cause analysis is a tool advocated by The Joint Commission when investigating sentinel events.

112) (B) HIPAA.

Patient information must remain protected. It can be discussed only on a need-to-know basis. It is protected by federal legislation, HIPAA. You often carry the patient's information on the requisition form. Still, you are not authorized to disclose it to anyone, even their close relatives, without the patient's written consent.

113) (B) Two.

When you encounter a difficult venipuncture, you can attempt another venipuncture either in another arm or below the first site. Always use a new needle. When the second attempt is not successful, do not try a third. Notify the nurse and request for another phlebotomist to collect the specimen.

114) (B) BUN.

Renal failure may progress as uremia, wherein blood contains too much urea and metabolic wastes. Blood urea nitrogen increases in uremia

115) (B) Cortisol and Cushing's disease.

Only Option B is correctly paired.

116) (D) Pancreatitis.

Pancreatitis causes excruciating abdominal pain from an inflammation of the pancreas. This may be due to excessive alcohol intake, gallbladder stones, cancer, or surgical complications. Although cholecystitis and cholangitis also cause abdominal pain from similar causes, the pain is colicky in nature and localized to the right upper quadrant.

117) (A) Pulmonary tuberculosis.

Tuberculosis is a contagious chronic infection due to *Mycobacterium tuberculosis*. It is among the notifiable diseases.

118) (D) Erythropoietin.

The kidneys also have endocrine functions. They produce erythropoietin, which signals the bone marrow to produce red blood cells.

119) (D) All of the above.

Sexually transmitted diseases cause inflammation or lesions in the genital organs. Common bacteria and their corresponding disease include:

- *Chlamydia trachomatis* (chlamydia)
- *Trichomonas vaginalis* (trichomoniasis)
- *Herpes simplex* virus (herpes genitalis)
- *Treponema pallidum* (syphilis)
- *Neisseria gonorrhea* (gonorrhea)

120) (A) Plasma.

Blood is about 55% plasma. When separated, it is clear and straw-colored. It is mostly water with some dissolved substances, such as proteins, vitamins, hormones, and wastes.

Test 4 Questions

1) A phlebotomist encounters an irate patient who refuses blood extraction. He threatens the patient that he will have someone hold him down. The phlebotomist is committing which of the following?

(A) Negligence.

(B) Defamation.

(C) Malpractice.

(D) Assault.

2) As a phlebotomist, you should always display professional behavior in the facility, such as which of the following?

(A) Keeping requisitions in disarray at the end of your shift; after all, the next shift can take care of it.

(B) Wearing a lot of cologne.

(C) Announcing your name with a smile as you enter the patient's room.

(D) Wearing an unwashed and wrinkled lab coat.

3) Being sensitive to cultural diversity is a desirable professional trait in the health care staff. A phlebotomist can respond appropriately by doing which of the following?

(A) Stereotyping patients.

(B) Asking politely first before proceeding with the venipuncture.

(C) Examining the patient's arm very quickly.

(D) Invading the patient's personal space.

4) Risk management aims to reduce risks to protect the interests of which of the following?

A) Patients.

B) Employers.

C) Healthcare staff.

D) All of the above.

5) As the Occupational Safety and Health Administration prescribes, the phlebotomist must wear which of the following?

(A) Dangling jewelry.

(B) Personal protective equipment.

(C) Long nail extensions.

(D) Hard hat and reflective gear.

6) Blood-borne pathogens may be transmitted through which of the following modes of exposure?

(A) Mucous membranes around the eyes.

(B) Lesions on the skin.

(C) Puncture from a used needle.

(D) All of the above.

7) The Centers for Disease Control and Prevention recommends hand hygiene in which of the following scenarios?

(A) Before performing an aseptic procedure (such as insertion of a catheter).

(B) Before touching a patient.

(C) After removing gloves.

(D) All of the above.

8) Which of the following is a disinfecting agent to clean surfaces contaminated with blood?

(A) Acetic acid.

(B) Sodium hypochlorite.

(C) Salicylic acid.

(D) Hydrogen peroxide.

9) Body systems are made up of a few organs that coordinate to perform interrelated functions. One example is which of the following?

(A) Integument.

(B) Muscle.

(C) Heart.

(D) Keratin.

10) The frontal lobe is located anterior to the parietal lobes of the brain. This means that the frontal lobe is which of the following?

(A) Beside the parietal lobes.

(B) Behind the parietal lobes.

(C) On the surface of the parietal lobes.

(D) At the front of the parietal lobes.

11) Which of the following planes cuts through vertically into equal right and left sections?

(A) Frontal.

(B) Sagittal.

(C) Midsagittal.

(D) Transverse.

12) The forearm is located distally from the arm. This means which of the following?

(A) The forearm is nearer to the center of the body than the arm.

(B) The forearm is farther from the center of the body than the arm.

(C) The forearm sits directly on the surface of the arm.

(D) The forearm is behind the arm.

13) Which of the following is an artery that runs along the lateral side of the wrist? A specific pulse is felt on the ventral surface of the wrist below the thumb.

(A) Radial.

(B) Carotid.

(C) Superior vena cava.

(D) Inferior vena cava.

14) Which of the following is not a vein in the antecubital fossa of the forearm?

(A) Median cubital.

(B) Cephalic.

(C) Bicipital.

(D) Basilic.

15) Which of the following is the process describing the formation of blood clots whenever a blood vessel is damaged?

(A) Hemostasis.

(B) Homeostasis.

(C) Hemophilia.

(D) Hemostat.

16) How do we determine a person's blood type?

(A) By conducting a blood transfusion procedure.

(B) By identifying how much blood a person has.

(C) By identifying the presence of antigens in the blood.

(D) By conducting a random antigen test.

17) Which of the following blood types is known as the universal receiver?

(A) A.

(B) B.

(C) AB.

(D) O.

18) Which of the following white blood cells is responsible for the histamine response during inflammatory processes?

(A) Eosinophil.

(B) Lymphocyte.

(C) Monocyte.

(D) Basophil.

19) Which of the following stages of hemostasis is being evaluated by a platelet count?

(A) Primary.

(B) Secondary.

(C) Fibrin clot.

(D) Clot lysis.

20) Which of the following stages of hemostasis is characterized by the retraction or tightening of the clot?

(A) Primary.

(B) Secondary.

(C) Fibrin clot.

(D) Clot lysis.

21) Which of the following conditions refers to an increase in the number of white blood cells, such as during infections?

(A) Leukemia.

(B) Leukocytosis.

(C) Polycythemia.

(D) Thrombocytosis.

22) Which of the following vessels is suitable for the exchange of nutrients, wastes, and gases?

(A) Veins.

(B) Arteries.

(C) Arterioles.

(D) Capillaries.

23) Which of the following needles has the largest diameter?

(A) 21-gauge.

(B) 18-gauge.

(C) 23-gauge.

(D) 16-gauge.

24) When are butterfly needles used for venipuncture

(A) Finger punctures.

(B) Dermal punctures.

(C) Adults with large veins.

(D) Adults with very small veins.

25) Skin cleansers are used to prevent bacterial contamination on the venipuncture sites. Which of the following antiseptics is better suited for blood culture collection?

(A) Povidone-iodine.

(B) 70% isopropyl alcohol.

(C) Soap and water.

(D) Sodium hypochlorite.

26) The purpose of the tourniquet in venipuncture is which of the following?

(A) To constrict arteries.

(B) To occlude blood flow to the veins.

(C) To make the veins harder.

(D) To collapse the veins.

27) Underfilling which of the following tubes leads to falsely elevated APTT levels?

(A) Lavender.

(B) Light green.

(C) Light blue.

(D) Yellow.

28) Which of the following information should be on a requisition form?

(A) Patient ID number.

(B) The requesting physician's name and signature.

(C) Test(s) requested.

(D) All of the above.

29) When meeting the patient, the phlebotomist is required to do which of the following?

(A) Describe the procedure using medical jargon to impress the patient.

(B) Inform the patient of the names of the tests to be done.

(C) Explain that they are going to collect specimens requested by the physician.

(D) Answer all the patient's questions about their condition.

30) You should position the patient's arm in which of the following ways to facilitate proper venipuncture?

(A) The elbow hyperextended.

(B) The arm downward and extended.

(C) The elbow bent at a 90° angle.

(D) The arms remaining at the side while the patient is standing.

31) You are about to draw blood for venipuncture from a seated patient when he tells you he is feeling a little lightheaded. You should do which of the following?

(A) Reassure him that the needle is very small; it should be painless.

(B) Act as though you did not hear him.

(C) Allow the patient tu lic down for the procedure.

(D) None of the above.

32) Which of the following is the best vein to use for venipuncture?

(A) Median cubital.

(B) Basilic.

(C) Cephalic.

(D) Axillary.

33) Which of the following is an indication of the use of tourniquets?

(A) It allows the veins to distend and helps with locating the venipuncture site.

(B) It makes blood collection easier, as blood has been allowed to pool.

(C) Both A and B.

(D) Neither A nor B.

34) All except which of the following describes correctly palpating a vein?

(A) Feeling for a pulse using the thumb.

(B) Feeling for depth.

(C) Feeling for the orientation of the vein.

(D) Feeling for a spongy and cylindrical surface using the index finger.

35) Which of the following is the proper way to cleanse the venipuncture site?

(A) Applying alcohol in a to-and-fro motion.

(B) Applying alcohol in a circular motion.

(C) Fanning the site to dry.

(C) Wiping the site with a cotton pad.

36) For a successful venipuncture procedure, you can prevent a vein from rolling by doing which of the following?

(A) Tightening the tourniquet.

(B) Keeping the skin taut by pulling it about one to 2 inches below and slightly lateral to the site.

(C) Anchoring the vein with your thumb and index finger above the site.

(D) Using a 25-gauge needle.

37) How should you discard the contaminated ETS and needle after venipuncture?

(A) Disassemble; discard needles in the sharps bin and the holder in the biohazard bin.

(B) Disassemble; discard needles in the sharps bin; keep the holder for the next patient.

(C) Discard the entire ETS needle and holder in the sharps bin.

(D) Recap the needle and dispose of it in the sharps bin.

38) How long is the ideal time for a coagulation assay specimen to reach the laboratory?

(A) 2 hours.

(B) 1 hour.

(C) 45 minutes.

(D) 30 minutes.

39) Which of the following statements on the consequences of improper transport is correct?

(A) Glycolysis causes falsely low blood glucose values.

(B) Hemolysis causes falsely low serum potassium values.

(C) Coagulation factors are not affected by storing at room temperature.

(D) Light does not affect bilirubin samples.

40) You arrive at a patient's room to do a routine venipuncture, but she is not in her bed. The nurse informs you that the patient was taken to the operating room an hour ago. Which of the following actions is appropriate?

(A) Find the patient in the operating room to draw the venipuncture.

(B) Postpone the procedure; leave the requisition with the nurses.

(C) Cancel the test and note it on the requisition slip.

(D) Inform the phlebotomy supervisor.

41) Which of the following statements is true regarding the removal of PPE?

(A) When removing PPE, the least contaminated items must be removed first.

(B) Do not touch the inside parts of the gloves and gowns.

(C) Discard each item of PPE as you remove it.

(D) After removing PPE, discard all items altogether.

42) Which of the following techniques may be employed to make the veins more prominent?

(A) Massage the patient's arm from the shoulder to the wrist.

(B) Apply a warm compress for 5 minutes.

(C) Apply a cold compress for 5 minutes.

(D) Briskly tap on the vein with your index fingers.

43) Pre-examination variables are those that affect the integrity of the specimens and alter test results. Which of the following statements is correct?

(A) Reference ranges are the same across age and sex.

(B) Pregnant women have decreased erythrocyte sedimentation counts.

(C) Smoking decreases hemoglobin and red cell count.

(D) TSH and cortisol levels are affected by the time of day.

44) Your patient fainted after you performed venipuncture at the outpatient laboratory. You should do which of the following?

(A) Use the spirit of ammonia to revive them.

(B) Recline and lower their head.

(C) Apply a warm compress to their forehead and nape.

(D) Restrain them.

45) Permission from the physician must be obtained when attempting to collect blood from which of the following?

(A) Pediatric patients.

(B) Diabetic patients.

(C) Lower-limb veins.

(D) Veins with IV fluid.

46) Which of the following is a potential complication when drawing blood on the arm on the same side as a recent mastectomy?

(A) Lymphedema.

(B) Sclerosis.

(C) Hemoconcentration.

(D) Hemolysis.

47) Which of the following is a suitable method for cleansing the site for an alcohol level blood test?

(A) Benzalkonium chloride.

(B) Sodium hypochlorite.

(C) 40% isopropyl alcohol.

(D) Premoistened tissues.

48) Which of the following can be the result of pulling a syringe plunger too hard and too fast?

(A) The specimen is hemoconcentrated.

(B) The vein collapses.

(C) The patient complains of an electric sensation.

(D) The patient bleeds longer.

49) Longer time may be required to apply pressure on which of the following patients?

(A) Hypertensive patients.

(B) Hemodialysis patients.

(C) Patients taking herbal medications.

(D) Obese patients.

50) Which of the following instances can cause a specimen to be rejected?

(A) Plasma with a reddish tint.

(B) Transporting a bilirubin specimen covered in foil.

(C) Incompletely filled SST.

(D) A clot forming in the red tube.

51) On which patient population is a dermal puncture appropriate?

(A) Neonates.

(B) Pediatric patients (up to 24 months old).

(C) Patients on glucose monitoring.

(D) All of the above.

52) Drawing too much blood from infants may cause which of the following:

(A) Iatrogenic anemia.

(B) Vasospasm.

(C) Infections.

(D) Inflammation.

53) Capillary blood contains lower levels of which of the following analytes?

(A) Potassium.

(B) Calcium.

(C) Protein.

(D) All of the above.

54) A dermal puncture that is too deep risks which of the following?

(A) Osteomyelitis.

(B) Osteoporosis.

(C) Osteochondritis.

(D) Both A and C.

55) Puncturing an improper site on the neonate's heel can cause which of the following?

(A) Additional agitation in the infant.

(B) Insufficient blood volume.

(C) Hemolysis.

(D) Accidental puncture of the calcaneus.

56) Which of the following is the optimal way to warm the heel before dermal puncture?

(A) Warm towel at 42° C for 5 minutes.

(B) Warm towel at 42° C for 15 minutes.

(C) Heel warmer for 2 minutes.

(D) Heel warmer for 10 minutes.

57) Which of the following techniques will allow you to collect more blood from a dermal puncture?

(A) Milking the site.

(B) Squeezing the site tightly.

(C) Applying alternating pressure.

(D) Performing multiple punctures.

58) Which of the following is a disease detected from a capillary blood sample blotted on a filter paper?

(A) Phenylketonuria.

(B) Hartnup disease.

(C) Malaria.

(D) Jaundice.

59) Collecting a newborn screen sample before the alcohol has completely dried causes which of the following?

(A) Inadequate sample.

(B) Serum rings to form.

(C) Diluted samples.

(D) Oversaturation.

60) Standard precautions are observed when preparing a peripheral blood smear. When does a blood smear first cease being infectious?

(A) When it has completely dried.

(B) When it is fixed with alcohol.

(C) When it is spread on the slide.

(D) When it has been autoclaved.

61) Which of the following refers to the presence of bacteria in the bloodstream?

(A) Sepsis.

(B) Bacteremia.

(C) Meningitis.

(D) Allergy.

62) When asked to collect a blood culture before giving STAT antibiotics, how should the blood sets be collected?

(A) Two sets of blood, 30 minutes apart.

(B) Two sets of blood; before and after antibiotics are started.

(C) At the same time, from one venipuncture site.

(D) At the same time, from two venipuncture sites.

63) When using a syringe collection system, which of the following is correct?

(A) The anaerobic bottle is filled first.

(B) The aerobic bottle is filled first.

(C) The volume of the blood to be collected is decreased.

(D) Either bottle can be filled first.

64) Which of the following is a suitable cleansing method before blood culture?

(A) Two-step method with chlorhexidine gluconate and povidone-iodine.

(B) Soaking the skin in a 2% tincture of iodine for 30 minutes.

(C) 70% isopropyl alcohol scrubbed in a circular motion, alone.

(D) ChloraPrep swabs to scrub the site using a to-and-fro motion, alone.

65) Which of the following is the correct blood culture volume requirement for children?

(A) 8 to 10 mL of blood per blood culture bottle.

(B) 1 mL for every 5 kg.

(C) 1 mL for every 5 pounds.

(D) Children who weigh over 25 kg; collect as much specimen as from an adult.

66) Specimens for which of the following tests are collected in 37° C tubes and should be kept warm?

(A) Warm agglutinins.

(B) Cryofibrinogen.

(C) Arterial blood gas.

(D) Bilirubin.

67) Specimens for which of the following tests should be collected in amber-colored bottles?

(A) Vitamin A.

(B) Vitamin B6.

(C) Vitamin B12.

(D) All of the above.

68) When collecting samples for blood alcohol levels, the site is ideally cleansed with which of the following?

(A) 70% isopropyl alcohol.

(B) Zephiran chloride.

(C) Povidone-iodine.

(D) ChloraPrep swabs.

69) Which of the following characteristics would make a volunteer not eligible to donate blood?

(A) 23 years old.

(B) Weight of 68 kg.

(C) Donated blood 10 weeks ago.

(D) A pulse rate of 115 bpm.

70) Donor units are routinely tested for the presence of which of the following blood-borne pathogens?

(A) *Trypanosoma cruzi.*

(B) *Treponema pallidum.*

(C) West Nile virus.

(D) All of the above.

71) The ideal skin cleansing procedure for donor blood collection involves which of the following?

(A) Two-step method with chlorhexidine gluconate and povidone-iodine.

(B) Two-step method with soap and water followed by chlorhexidine gluconate or povidone-iodine.

(C) 70% isopropyl alcohol scrubbed in a circular motion for 30 seconds.

(D) ChloraPrep swabs to scrub the site using a to-and-fro motion for 30 seconds.

72) Following successful blood donation, volunteers should be instructed to do which of the following?

(A) Drink plenty of fluids.

(B) Avoid strenuous activities.

(C) Remove the bandage after 4 hours.

(D) All of the above.

73) The volume of urine required for drug testing is which of the following?

(A) 15 to 30 mL of urine.

(B) 20 to 25 mL of urine.

(C) 30 to 45 mL of urine.

(D) 35 to 50 mL of urine.

74) The volume of blood collected in a blood bag is which of the following?

(A) 305 to 395 mL.

(B) 405 to 495 mL.

(C) 450 to 500 mL.

(D) 350 to 400 mL.

75) All except which of the following statements regarding semen collection are true?

(A) Taking note of the time of collection is necessary.

(B) The patient should refrain from sexual activity for 3 days.

(C) The sample should be collected only in the laboratory.

(D) Condoms are not suitable for semen collection.

76) The correct method of collecting a throat swab involves which of the following?

(A) Directing the swab straight to the back of the throat.

(B) Directing the swab to the cheeks, tongue, and back of the throat.

(C) Avoiding areas with inflammation or ulceration.

(D) All of the above.

77) Which of the following specimens may be used to investigate hemolytic disease or genetic disease or ascertain fetal lung maturity?

(A) Amniotic fluid.

(B) Synovial fluid.

(C) Cerebrospinal fluid.

(D) Serous fluid.

78) For CSF collection, the needle is inserted at this level of the lumbar vertebrae:

(A) Between L1 and L2.

(B) Between L2 and L3.

(C) Between L4 and L5.

(D) Between L5 and L6.

79) Which of the following statements is correct?

(A) Tubes for chemistry and immunology are kept at room temperature.

(B) Tubes for microbiology are refrigerated.

(C) Tubes for hematology should be analyzed within 1 hour.

(D) Tubes for cytology are frozen.

80) Which of the following type of serous fluid is increased by tuberculosis?

(A) Pleural.

(B) Pericardial.

(C) Parietal.

(D) Peritoneal.

81) When is the best time to collect sputum?

(A) Right after a meal.

(B) Right after waking up in the morning.

(C) Right before going to bed.

(D) Right after smoking.

82) Detection of *H. pylori* from the breath involves which of the following?

(A) *H. pylori* produces carbonase, which degrades C-urea.

(B) The patient ingests C-urea, which is a radioactive carbon isotope.

(C) Hydrogen level is serially measured every 15 minutes over 3 to 5 hours.

(D) Increased carbon dioxide level in the second sample indicates *H. pylori* infection.

83) Which of the following refers to a part of a specimen transferred to another tube?

(A) Serum.

(B) Plasma.

(C) Buffy coat.

(D) Aliquot.

84) Which of the following is the ideal temperature for storing serum or plasma, which cannot be tested after 8 hours?

(A) 27° C.

(B) 10° C.

(C) -20° C.

(D) 7° C.

85) For how long can an APTT specimen remain at room temperature?

(A) 2 hours.

(B) 4 hours.

(C) 8 hours.

(D) 24 hours.

86) For how long can reticulocyte count specimens in EDTA tubes be refrigerated?

(A) 12 hours.

(B) 24 hours.

(C) 48 hours.

(D) 72 hours.

87) Which of the following categories of infectious substances does *Bacillus anthracis* fall under?

(A) Category A.

(B) Category B.

(C) Category C.

(D) Category D.

88) When shipping laboratory specimens, the label “Class 9 miscellaneous” indicates which of the following?

(A) The contents are Category A.

(B) The contents are Category B.

(C) The contents are packed in dry ice.

(D) The contents are packed with refrigerant packs.

89) Which of the following is a series of black-and-white lines that facilitate data entry by automatically inputting information?

(A) Barcodes.

(B) Radiofrequency ID.

(C) Silicon chips.

(D) CPT codes.

90) Which of the following procedures utilizes complex instrumentation and interpretation that requires higher levels of understanding? The performance of these tests is subjected to proficiency testing. An example is blood culture and antibiotic sensitivity testing.

(A) Waived test.

(B) Provider-performed microscopy.

(C) Moderate complexity.

(D) High complexity.

91) Which of the following is a high-complexity test?

(A) Urine pregnancy test.

(B) Glycosylated hemoglobin test.

(C) Blood culture and sensitivity.

(D) Complete blood count.

92) Which of the following organizations inspects laboratories regularly to ensure they comply with the standards?

(A) CLIA.

(B) CMS.

(C) OSHA.

(D) CAP.

93) When performing tests from a new shipment of test kits, you should do which of the following?

(A) Read the enclosed instructions.

(B) Discard the enclosed instructions.

(C) Refer to the old instructions posted on your workspace.

(D) Ask your supervisor.

94) An internal or procedural control determines which of the following?

(A) Whether a test is working properly.

(B) Whether the electronic functions of the equipment are working properly.

(C) Whether the sample size is adequate.

(D) All of the above.

95) Quality control ascertains the correctness of test results. Which of the following situations prompts quality-control testing?

(A) When a test shows an invalid result.

(B) After a power outage.

(C) After hiring new staff to perform the test.

(D) All of the above.

96) A waived testing can be performed on which of the following samples?

(A) Whole blood.

(B) Urine.

(C) Saliva.

(D) All of the above.

97) Improperly timing a test leads to false results. Reading a result after the indicated time causes an invalid result under which of the following conditions?

(A) Test sample and reagent have not completed their chemical reaction.

(B) Colors underdevelop or are faded.

(C) The reaction moves beyond the visible window.

(D) Colors overdevelop.

98) Which of the following is a test result that demands the immediate attention of the physician?

(A) Red flag.

(B) Panic value.

(C) Abnormal results.

(D) STAT test.

99) A positive test result for which of the following conditions requires mandatory reporting to public health authorities?

(A) Notifiable disease.

(B) Confirmatory test.

(C) Critical values.

(D) Quality-control test.

100) When a patient does not respond to stimuli, such as loud noise, shaking, or pinching their earlobe, the phlebotomist should attempt which of the following?

(A) A sternal rub.

(B) A needle prick.

(C) Chest compressions.

(D) Calling for help.

101) Which of the following lists the correct order of steps for an initial survey?

(A) Call for help and check the patient's airway and breathing.

(B) Call for help, begin chest compressions and check airway and breathing.

(C) Call for help, check for bleeding and check airway and breathing.

(D) Check airway and breathing, call for help, and begin compressions.

102) The depth of chest compressions in infants should be:

(A) 1.5 inches.

(B) 1.5 cm.

(C) 2 inches.

(D) 2 cm.

103) Which of the following statements regarding cardiopulmonary resuscitation in infants is correct?

(A) Place two fingers on the infant's sternum, just below the level of the nipples.

(B) Using the heel of one hand, push on the sternum to depress it at least 2 inches.

(C) The rate should be in a range of 110 to 160 per minute.

(D) All of the above.

104) Which of the following should a phlebotomist perform when receiving a new shipment of evacuated tubes?

(A) Quality management.

(B) Quality assessment.

(C) Quality systems essentials.

(D) Quality control.

105) The National Patient Safety Goals of the Laboratory include which of the following?

(A) Three-method verification for accurately identifying the patient.

(B) Labeling specimen containers immediately after leaving the patient.

(C) Informing the right staff of critical values.

(D) All of the above.

106) A new phlebotomist has forgotten to extract a routine serum electrolyte test on one patient. A nurse brought this to the laboratory's attention when the test was missing from the reported results. The laboratory should do which of the following?

(A) Fire the phlebotomist.

(B) Repeat the venipuncture during the next sweep.

(C) Immediately perform the test as STAT.

(D) Make up the results.

107) Which of the following is correct when documenting in the patient's chart?

(A) Writing using a pencil.

(B) Using your own abbreviation.

(C) Deleting electronic records.

(D) Signing your initials with the date and time of collection.

108) Which of the following is the main goal of quality-management systems?

(A) Reduce medical errors.

(B) Improve employee working conditions.

(C) Increase efficiency.

(D) All of the above.

109) Which of the following evaluate quality systems essentials in phlebotomy?

(A) Quality indicators.

(B) Quality assessment.

(C) Quality management.

(D) Quality control.

110) Which of the following systems involved in quality management aims to reduce errors to the acceptable level of 3.4 defects for every million opportunities?

(A) Lean system.

(B) Six Sigma.

(C) Root cause analysis.

(D) Nonconforming events.

111) The root cause analysis focuses on which of the following?

(A) Failures of the phlebotomist.

(B) Failures of the physician.

(C) Failures of the patient.

(D) Failures of the process.

112) Which of the following laboratory tests is paired with its correct clinical correlation?

(A) Calcium and liver disease.

(B) Cortisol and acromegaly.

(C) Pap smear and pregnancy.

(D) Albumin and malnutrition.

113) Which of the following conditions causes hypercalcemia from excessive bone resorption?

(A) Hyperthyroidism.

(B) Hyperparathyroidism.

(C) Hypothyroidism.

(D) Hypoparathyroidism.

114) Which of the following hormones help maintain the pregnancy?

(A) Progesterone.

(B) Estrogen.

(C) Human beta chorionic gonadotropin.

(D) Only A and C.

115) Which of the following bacteria is correctly paired with the sexually transmitted disease it can cause?

(A) *Chlamydia trachomatis* (gonorrhea).

(B) *Treponema pallidum* (herpes).

(C) *Trichomonas vaginalis* (syphilis).

(D) *Neisseria gonorrhea* (gonorrhea).

116) A phlebotomist is not allowed to remain at work until they are out of the infectious stage of which of the following diseases?

(A) Gonorrhea.

(B) Streptococcal tonsilitis.

(C) Acute gastroenteritis.

(D) Chlamydia.

117) Which of the following bacteria arises from antibiotic overuse and colonizes the intestines, causing toxic megacolon?

(A) *Clostridium tetani.*

(B) *Clostridium botulinum.*

(C) *Clostridium difficile.*

(D) All of the above.

118) Which of the following conditions causes joint pain and swelling, erythema, and warmth of the overlying skin?

(A) Fracture.

(B) Osteoporosis.

(C) Arthralgia.

(D) Arthritis.

119) Which of the following conditions results from abnormal transmission of electrical impulses in the brain and may rarely be triggered by venipuncture?

(A) Stroke.

(B) Bell's palsy.

(C) Seizure.

(D) Amyotrophic lateral sclerosis.

120) There are no vaccines for all except which of the following blood-borne pathogens?

(A) Hepatitis B.

(B) HIV.

(C) Hepatitis C.

(D) HTLV-1.

Test 4 Answers and Explanations

1) (D) Assault.

Assault refers to touching another person or threatening to do so without their consent. For example, when dealing with an irate patient, the phlebotomist threatens to hold him down to extract blood. When a patient refuses to have blood extracted even after you have explained it, you must accept the patient's wishes, inform the nurses in charge, and document the patient's refusal on your request form.

2) (C) Announcing your name with a smile as you enter the patient's room.

Most of your duties center around the patient. Always be aware that they are often sick and anxious. Always introduce yourself before you approach the patient. This approach also helps you ask the patient's name to identify them. Keeping requisitions in disarray (A) and wearing an unwashed lab coat (D) demonstrate sloppiness, which reflects as sloppiness with work. Wearing a lot of cologne (C) is a disregard for others, who may be hypersensitive to strong smells.

3) (B) Asking politely first before proceeding with the venipuncture.

Respecting cultural diversity aids in communication and demonstrates professionalism. For example, a Muslim woman or her husband may not allow a male phlebotomist to extract her blood. Asking politely first and accommodating their culture will demonstrate professionalism. Stereotyping patients (A), examining them very quickly and without consent (C), and invading the patient's personal space (D) are disrespectful actions and do not portray good professional traits.

4) (D) All of the above.

Risk management aims to develop protocols to protect everyone—patients (A) and health care staff (C)—from preventable harm. Employers (B) are protected as well, as they can avoid the costs that harm might accrue.

5) (B) Personal protective equipment.

OSHA has implemented guidelines designed to prevent infections from spreading across healthcare facilities by regulating the use of personal protective equipment, or PPE. Wearing dangling jewelry (A) and nail extensions (C) are avoided. While a hard hat and reflective gear (D) are protective equipment, wearing these in the laboratory is unnecessary.

6) (D) All of the above.

Accidental needlestick injuries are the most common BBP exposures. As a rule of thumb, never recap a needle. Use needle safety devices. Dispose of all sharps into appropriate containers immediately. Never reach into these when disposing of sharps. Additionally, blood-borne pathogens may utilize the mucous membranes around the eyes or lesions on the skin as portals of entry. Masks and eye protection are important components of PPE.

7) (D) All of the above.

Crucial moments for handwashing as recommended by the CDC include:

- Before entering a patient's immediate environment
- Before carrying out an aseptic procedure, such as the insertion of an indwelling catheter
- After leaving a patient's bed, room, or ward
- After handling bodily fluids (i.e., blood) or any contaminated surfaces
- After removing gloves

8) (B) Sodium hypochlorite .

In the event of spills on equipment and surfaces, blood or fluids are first removed with an absorbent material. Do not mop or wipe it off. The area is then disinfected with sodium hypochlorite (1 part diluted in 10 parts water).

9) (A) Integument.

The integumentary system is the largest organ system of the human body. It is composed of the skin and its associated glands, along with the hair and nails.

The muscle (B) and keratin (D) are both types of tissue, while the heart is an organ (C).

10) (D) At the front of the parietal lobes.

The directional term *anterior* was used, which describes the structure to be preceding or directly in front of another. Therefore, the frontal lobe lies in front of the parietal lobes

11) (C) Midsagittal.

The human body is described across different planes. The midsagittal plane cuts through vertically into equal right and left sections.

12) (B) The forearm is farther from the center of the body than the arm.

The directional term *distal* was used, describing something farther from the center of the body. Therefore, the forearm is farther from the body's center than the arm.

13) (A) Radial.

The radial artery runs along the lateral area of the wrist. Its pulse is felt on the ventral surface right below the thumb. The carotid artery is a large artery branching near the aorta, while the superior and inferior vena cava are veins.

14) (C) Bicipital.

There is no bicipital vein found in the antecubital fossa of the forearm. Rather, a bicipital aponeurosis separates the superficial from the deeper structures in the fossa. All other choices are veins that branch off the dorsal venous plexus of the hands.

15) (A) Hemostasis.

Hemostasis refers to the formation of blood clots in response to a blood vessel injury. Option B: Homeostasis is the clinical term for equilibrium. Option C: Hemophilia is a blood dyscrasia resulting from lacking factor VIII or IX. Option D: Hemostat is a device that clamps the blood bag tubing.

16) (C) By identifying the presence of antigens in the blood.

The erythrocytes can be coated with antigens. These determine a person's blood type. It can either be A, B, or AB, depending on which antigen is present. The O blood type contains no antigens.

17) (C) AB.

Type AB is considered the universal receiver. The receiver's plasma has neither anti-A nor anti-B antibodies; thus, it cannot form a transfusion reaction with the donor's blood cells.

18) (D) Basophil.

Basophils are few and sometimes absent at 0% to 1% of the total leukocytes. They are responsible for the histamine response during inflammatory processes. They also contain granules of heparin to prevent blood clots.

19) (A) Primary.

A platelet count is ordered to determine whether the patient adequately forms a platelet plug during this stage of hemostasis. The primary stage of hemostasis occurs immediately after an injury. The vasculature constricts to prevent blood from leaking out. Platelets aggregate and clump (aggregation). They adhere to the injured area (adhesion) as a temporary plug.

20) (C) Fibrin clot.

The cascade ends after factor XIII is activated. At this point, the fibrin clot is stabilized, and the clot retracts or tightens.

21) (B) Leukocytosis.

Leukocytosis refers to an increase in the number of white blood cells, such as during infections. Option A is a type of cancer resulting from a dysregulated increase of leukocytes. Option C refers to the abnormal increase in the levels of erythrocytes or hematocrit. Option D refers to an increase in platelets.

22) (D) Capillaries.

Capillary beds in the tissues are suitable for the exchange of nutrients, wastes, and gases. The arteries carry oxygenated blood, while the veins carry deoxygenated blood.

23) (D) 16-gauge.

Needle gauge refers to the diameter of the needle and is indicated by a number from 16 to 25. A lower number indicates a thicker needle, while a higher number indicates a thinner needle.

24) (D) Adults with very small veins.

Winged blood collection sets are also called "butterflies." These are routinely used for IV infusions and venipuncture in smaller and very fragile veins, such as in cancer patients, small children, and geriatric patients.

25) (A) Povidone-iodine.

Skin cleansers, such as 70% isopropyl alcohol, avoid bacterial contamination during specimen collection. For blood cultures, stronger solutions are required, such as povidone-iodine or, if allergic to this, chlorhexidine. Remember to ask for a history of allergy to either substance.

26) (B) To occlude blood flow to the veins.

A tourniquet is a band of flat, disposable vinyl or nitrile applied around a limb. Its purpose is to occlude blood flow through the veins but not through an artery. This allows superficial veins to distend and become more palpable.

27) (C) Light blue.

An underfilled light-blue tube causes a false elevation of APTT due to a wrong blood-to-citrate ratio.

28) (D) All of the above.

The following information should always be on the requisition form:

- Patient identifiers: full name, age, gender, and birth date; location
- Patient ID number (assigned by the hospital or the laboratory)
- The requesting physician's name and signature
- Test(s) requested
- Date and time of collection
- Urgency—whether STAT, routine, or a timed collection
- Other information—billing codes or ICD codes, special patient information (allergy to latex, fasting, areas to avoid for use in venipuncture)

29) (C) Explain that they are going to collect specimens requested by the physician.

When meeting the patient, greet them with a smile. Give them your name, and explain that you are there to collect specimens requested by the patient's physician. If questioned about which tests are requested and why, politely inform the patient that this information is best given by their physician.

30) (B) The arm is downward and extended.

The correct position of the patient's arm should be downward and extended. This way, your tubes may fill properly and avoid additive carryover. Do not hyperextend their elbows. This may make it difficult to find the veins.

31) (C) Allow the patient to lie down for the procedure.

While it is important to reassure the patient throughout the procedure, never promise that it will be painless. Stay alert to the patient's condition, as some patients may faint at any time. If the patient lets you know that they may faint, have them lie down for the venipuncture. Importantly, ensure the seats have barriers that can catch a falling patient. If you lowered a bed rail during the venipuncture procedure, always return it before leaving the patient.

32) (A) Median cubital.

The median cubital is the preferred venipuncture site since it is larger and well-anchored. It lies in the center of the antecubital area. It is the least painful site, since this vein overlies aponeurosis.

33) (C) Both A and B.

A tourniquet allows the veins to distend by obstructing venous return. It is not strong enough to impede arteries. This helps with locating the venipuncture site and makes blood collection easier, as blood has been allowed to pool. Following this principle, you first use the tourniquet to choose your venipuncture site. CLSI recommends waiting at least 2 minutes before reapplying it to draw blood.

34) (A) Feeling for a pulse using the thumb.

After applying the tourniquet, your index finger finds veins on sight or palpates. Veins feel rubbery or spongy and cylindrical. You can feel the vein's direction or orientation and depth. Unlike arteries, veins should not have a pulse. The thumb is not suitable for palpating a vein, since it has its own pulse.

35) (A) Applying alcohol in a to-and-fro motion.

Routinely, 70% isopropyl alcohol on a presoaked pad is used to prepare the site for the venipuncture. Rub 2 to 3 inches around the venipuncture site in a to-and-fro motion. You may need to repeat this with a new alcohol pad if the patient's arm is still visibly soiled.

36) (B) Keeping the skin taut by pulling it about 1 to 2 inches below and slightly lateral to the site.

To perform venipuncture, position the needle with the bevel up. With the thumb of your non-dominant hand, pull the skin about 1 to 2 inches below and slightly lateral to the site. This keeps it taut around the selected vein. It helps to keep the vein firmly in place and prevents it from rolling. Do not anchor the vein with your thumb and index finger above the site. Any sudden movement, especially in a noncooperative patient, can cause accidental needle pricks on these fingers.

37) (C) Discard the entire ETS needle and holder in the sharps bin.

Do not disassemble the blood collection systems. Discard the entire used ETS needle and holder into the sharps container.

38) (C) 45 minutes.

Tubes with anticoagulant additives must be centrifuged within 2 hours. The ideal time for the specimen to reach the laboratory department should be within 45 minutes. This allows time for immediate centrifugation.

39) (A) Glycolysis causes falsely low blood glucose values.

Glucose determinations are affected by glycolysis, which causes falsely low values. Option B: Hemolysis causes falsely high potassium values. Option C: Coagulation factors may be labile to temperature. Option D: Bilirubin is photosensitive.

40) (B) Postpone the procedure; leave the requisition with the nurses.

Patients may not be in their room when you arrive for venipuncture. Locate them through the nurse. They may just be walking around or taken to radiology or other units.

If you need to draw blood for a timed specimen or a STAT test, it may be necessary to go to the unit where the patient was taken. In this case, the test is routine. It is not necessary to go to the unit. The most appropriate action would be to inform the nurse to reschedule the test or alert the laboratory when the patient is available. Note this appropriately on the requisition form.

41) (C) Discard each item of PPE as you remove it.

When removing PPE, the most contaminated items must be removed first, not the least contaminated. Touch only the inside parts of the gloves and gowns, ensuring the contaminated areas do not touch your skin. Discard each item of PPE as you remove it.

42) (B) Apply a warm compress for 5 minutes.

Techniques to make the veins more prominent:

- Massage the patient's forearm, moving up from the wrist to the elbow.
- Ask the patient to hang their arm down the side of the chair briefly.
- Apply a warm compress to the area for about 5 minutes.

43) (D) TSH and cortisol levels are affected by the time of day.

Thyroid-stimulating hormones and cortisol levels are notably sensitive to diurnal variations. These levels can be about 50% different between an 8 a.m. sample and a 4 p.m. sample. Option A: Reference ranges are affected by age and sex. Option B: Pregnancy is a pro-inflammatory state, which may also increase erythrocyte sedimentation rates and certain clotting factors. Option C: Prolonged effects of nicotine include hemoconcentration and lower immunoglobulin levels.

44) (B) Recline and lower their head.

When your patient has fainted, immediately release the tourniquet. Withdraw the needle and apply pressure to the venipuncture site. While doing this, call for help. In the outpatient setting, recline the patient and lower their head. Be careful that they do not fall.

45) (C) Lower-limb veins.

When no other arm or hand veins are suitable, the lower-limb veins can be used. Obtain permission from the physician first. These veins are more prone to infections and thrombi.

46) (A) Lymphedema.

Venipuncture on the arm on the side of a recent mastectomy potentially causes lymphedema, since lymph nodes may have been dissected during mastectomy, and lymphatic circulation is obstructed.

47) (A) Benzalkonium chloride.

When collecting samples for blood alcohol levels, the site is cleansed with solutions other than 70% isopropyl alcohol. This may be soap and water or benzalkonium (Zephiran) chloride.

48) (B) The vein collapses.

The vein collapses when exerting too much pressure on it, such as by a syringe plunger pulled too hard or too fast.

49) (C) Patients taking herbal medications.

It is prudent to ask your patients, especially the elderly, about the use of blood thinners and herbal medications. This will indicate the need for more pressure. When there is excess bleeding after applying 5 minutes of adequate pressure, you may need to ask your patient if they have been taking herbal medications. Bleeding is a common adverse effect of herbal medicine. It should be noted on the requisitions.

50) (A) Plasma with a reddish tint.

Plasma with a pink or reddish tint is a sign of hemolysis. Tests cannot be run on these specimens and should be rejected. Option B: Bilirubin is photosensitive and should remain covered in foil. Option C: SST tubes are not affected by the fill level. Option D: Clots are expected to form in a plain red tube.

51) (B) Pediatric patients (up to 24 months old).

Dermal puncture is preferable for infants (24 months old and below) with lower blood volume and often no suitable superficial veins. Burn patients, chemotherapy patients, the elderly, those on glucose monitoring, and patients with scarred and inaccessible veins may benefit from dermal punctures.

52) (A) Iatrogenic anemia.

In newborns, the blood extracted should not exceed 3% of their blood volume at any given time and should not exceed 10% of their blood volume in one month.

53) (D) All of the above.

Capillary blood contains a higher glucose level and lower potassium, calcium, and protein levels than venous blood. Be sure to make a note when dermal puncture was performed to alert the physicians as they interpret the test results.

54) (D) Both A and C.

The main concern when performing dermal punctures is to avoid puncturing the bone. This can lead to bone infections (osteomyelitis) or inflammation (osteochondritis).

55) (D) Accidental puncture of the calcaneus.

Suitable areas for heel punctures are on the bottom of the heel, at either the medial or lateral surfaces. These areas provide the most space from the skin to the calcaneus bone. The main concern when performing dermal punctures is to avoid puncturing the bone. This can lead to bone infections (osteomyelitis) or inflammation (osteochondritis).

56) (A) Warm towel at 42° C for 5 minutes.

Applying a warm washcloth at 42° Celsius or a heel warmer for about 3 to 5 minutes (but less than 10 minutes) is effective in warming the area without affecting the test results. Be careful not to cause burns, especially in very young children.

57) (C) Applying alternating pressure.

Gently applying and then releasing pressure about half an inch away from the area will allow for better blood flow. Do not milk the area; this will only contaminate the sample with tissue fluid. Squeezing the site tightly constricts blood flow. Performing multiple punctures causes additional discomfort to the patient. Always aim to collect enough specimens from a single puncture by following the proper procedures.

58) (A) Phenylketonuria.

To perform newborn screening tests, blood from the heel puncture is blotted on an area marked by circles on the specimen card. Current laboratory assays may detect as many as 50 of these conditions. The required specific screening varies with each state. Regardless, all states include screening for cystic fibrosis, phenylketonuria, galactosemias, and congenital hypothyroidism.

59) (B) Serum rings to form.

The choices describe instances when a newborn screening card may be rejected, but collecting from an area contaminated with wet alcohol causes only the formation of serum rings on the sample. The other choices are caused by other factors, such as applying excess blood or improper techniques.

60) (B) When it is fixed with alcohol.

Be sure to wear your gloves throughout the peripheral blood smear preparation. The specimen is potentially infectious until it has been fixed in alcohol.

61) (B) Bacteremia.

Bacteremia is the presence of bacteria in the bloodstream. *Sepsis* is the clinical term used when the patient has a systemic inflammation (such as fever and increased heart rate; or increased white cell counts) along with bacteremia.

62) (D) At the same time, from two venipuncture sites.

When an antibiotic is to be started immediately, a blood culture may be requested as STAT at the emergency department just before the antibiotics are given. In this case, you will simultaneously draw both blood culture sets from different venipuncture sites.

63) (A) The anaerobic bottle is filled first.

When the specimen has been collected in a syringe, the anaerobic bottle (red blood culture bottle) is inoculated first. This prevents exposure to air, which can destroy anaerobic bacteria.

64) (D) ChloraPrep swabs to scrub the site using a to-and-fro motion, alone.

Of the choices, only ChloraPrep swabs are the correct method of cleansing the skin.

65) (B) 1 mL for every 5 kg.

Pediatric bottles are available for use on children. The volume of blood collected is computed based on the child's weight. A sufficient sample is 1 mL for every 5 kg (or 10 pounds).

66) (B) Cryofibrinogen.

Cold agglutinins, cryofibrinogen, and cryoglobulin should be kept warm.

67) (D) All of the above.

Photosensitive analytes deteriorate upon exposure to light or ultraviolet radiation. These specimens may be wrapped in aluminum foil or collected in amber-colored tubes. Photosensitive analytes include bilirubin, vitamin A, porphyrins, folate, niacin (vitamin B6), and cyanocobalamin (vitamin B12).

68) (B) Zephiran chloride.

When collecting samples for blood alcohol levels, the site is cleansed with solutions other than 70% isopropyl alcohol. This may be soap and water or benzalkonium (Zephiran) chloride.

69) (D) A pulse rate of 115 bpm.

A pulse rate of 115 bpm is too high and may be attributed to underlying infections or conditions, making it unsafe for a volunteer to donate blood. The eligibility criteria for blood donation requires volunteers to be at least 17 years old (A), at least 50 kg (B), afebrile, with a normal blood pressure above 90/50 but below 180/100 mmHg, and a pulse rate of 50 to 100 bpm. At least 8 weeks should have passed since a volunteer's last blood donation, which makes 10 weeks (C) adequate time for a person's stores of blood cells to be replenished.

70) (D) All of the above.

Donor screening also involves testing a sample of their blood for ABO and Rh blood type and testing for the presence of blood-borne pathogens. Donor units are tested for *Trypanosoma cruzi, Treponema pallidum,* HIV, hepatitis B and C, HTLV, and West Nile virus.

71) (B) Two-step method with soap and water followed by chlorhexidine gluconate or povidone-iodine.

Adequate skin cleansing for donor blood requires two steps. First, by soap and water or a detergent scrub, then by application of iodine or chlorhexidine gluconate. Allow at least 30 seconds for the cleansers to dry before proceeding.

72) (D) All of the above.

Post-donation care involves confirming that the bleeding has stopped and bandaging the site. Instruct the donors that these can be removed after 4 hours. Allow donors to have some juice or snacks before leaving the blood collection center. They should be instructed to drink plenty of fluids and avoid strenuous activities or heavy lifting during the day.

73) (C) 30 to 45 mL of urine.

An adequate sample for drug testing is 30 to 45 ml of urine.

74) (B) 405 to 495 mL.

The blood bag contains citrate-phosphate-dextrose or citrate-phosphate-dextrose-adenine to preserve the blood and prevent clots. It is designed to collect 405 to 495 milliliters of blood.

75) (C) The sample should be collected only in the laboratory.

Ideally, the sample should be collected in the laboratory, but patients may choose to collect the sample at home. When doing so, it is important to provide him with clear and written instructions.

76) (A) Directing the swab straight to the back of the throat.

When performing a throat swab, direct the swab straight to the back of the throat. Be sure to swab areas with inflammation or ulceration. Do not touch the cheeks, teeth, or lips throughout this process.

77) (A) Amniotic fluid.

The unborn fetus lies within the amniotic fluid. Physicians may aspirate a sample of this to investigate hemolytic disease or genetic disease or ascertain fetal lung maturity.

78) (C) Between L4 and L5.

Collection of CSF is done by a physician through a lumbar puncture procedure. A needle is inserted between the L3, L4, and L5 lumbar vertebrae. In these areas, it is possible to collect the fluid without damaging the spinal cord.

79) (C) Tubes for hematology should be analyzed within 1 hour.

CSF tests are always regarded as STAT specimens because cells begin deteriorating within the first hour. The tubes for chemistry and immunology may be refrigerated. Tubes for microbiology and hematology are kept at room temperature since fastidious microorganisms (e.g., *Neisseria meningitides*) cannot survive at lower temperatures.

80) (A) Pleural.

Pleural fluid increases in pulmonary conditions, such as tuberculosis, lung infections, and tumors. This is known as pleural effusion.

81) (B) Right after waking up in the morning.

The first-morning sample is ideal to ensure a large enough collection. Patients are instructed to collect the samples before a meal and without smoking. Moments before expectorating sputum, have the patient gargle with water (but do not swallow) to obtain a sample with the least contamination.

82) (D) Increased carbon dioxide level in the second sample indicates *H. pylori* infection.

In the C-urea breath test, the levels of exhaled carbon dioxide from both balloons are compared. An increase in the second sample indicates infection with *H. pylori*. Option A: *H. pylori* produces urease, not carbonase. Option B: C-urea is a carbon isotope that is not radioactive. Option C: Hydrogen levels are measured in the hydrogen breath test.

83) (D) Aliquot.

An aliquot refers to the part of a specimen transferred to another tube.

84) (D) 7° C.

Refrigerated serum or plasma should be maintained at 2° C to 8° C if testing is not done after 8 hours. It can be kept for up to 48 hours.

85) (B) 4 hours.

APTT specimen may remain at room temperature for up to 4 hours.

86) (D) 72 hours.

Reticulocytes should be counted from 6 hours of collection in EDTA tubes kept at room temperature. Refrigeration may extend this limit up to 72 hours.

87) (A) Category A.

Biohazardous material may be designated one of two classifications. Category A: Exposure to these substances may be potentially disabling or life-threatening to humans (UN 2814) or animals—for instance, *Bacillus anthracis.*

88) (C) The contents are packed in dry ice.

Frozen samples should be packed in dry ice with an additional label indicating "Class 9 miscellaneous."

89) (A) Barcodes.

This is a system of data entry that automatically inputs information by means of scanning unique black-and-white lines. This method decreases the possibility of making clerical errors.

90) (D) High complexity.

These procedures utilize complex instrumentation. Interpretation requires higher levels of understanding, and the performance of these tests is subjected to proficiency testing

91) (C) Blood culture and sensitivity.

High-complexity procedures utilize complex instrumentation. Interpretation requires higher levels of understanding, and the performance of these tests is subjected to proficiency testing (e.g., blood culture and sensitivity)

92) (B) CMS.

The Center for Medicare & Medicaid Service (CMS) or accredited agencies regularly inspect laboratories to ensure they comply with the CLIA standards.

93) (A) Read the enclosed instructions.

Always read the enclosed instructions for any changes when receiving a new lot of test kits or a new shipment. Inform your colleagues and supervisor if there are any.

94) (D) All of the above.

An internal or procedural control determines whether a test is working properly, the sample size is adequate, and, when applicable, the electronic functions of the equipment are in proper working conditions.

95) (D) All of the above.

Quality controls are scheduled regularly with consideration to the following:

- Manufacturer instructions
- When checking the validity of the test
- After environmental changes (such as electrical outages and refrigerator issues)
- For every trainee or new personnel who will be performing the test
- With every shipment of test kits or test reagents

96) (D) All of the above.

Waived tests should be done only on unprocessed samples, such as:

- Whole blood
- Anticoagulated blood
- Urine
- Feces
- Swabs from either the throat or nasopharynx
- Salivary fluids
- Gastric tissue biopsy

97) (C) The reaction moves beyond the visible window.

Reading a result after the indicated time leads to an invalid test when the reaction moves beyond the visible window on the test cassette.

98) (B) Panic value.

Critical or panic values are results that need the physician's immediate attention.

99) (A) Notifiable disease.

Public health agencies have flagged certain diseases as "notifiable." Testing sites are required to report confirmed positive or reactive results for infectious diseases, such as COVID-19, tuberculosis, active hepatitis, anthrax, and botulism, among others.

100) (A) A sternal rub.

If it is difficult to rouse a patient, try making a loud noise, shaking them, or pinching their earlobe. If they do not respond, elicit pain by performing a sternal rub.

101) (A) Call for help and check the patient's airway and breathing.

If the patient is unresponsive, call for help immediately. Do not leave the patient. Perform the initial survey while waiting for help to arrive. Check the patient's airway by tilting their chin slightly upward and opening the mouth. If something is lodged, position the patient on their side and remove the obstruction. Otherwise, check for breathing by listening for breath sounds next to the patient's mouth and simultaneously watching their chest for movement. If the patient is unresponsive and not breathing, immediately begin chest compressions.

102) (A) 1.5 inches.

To perform chest compressions on infants, place two fingers on the infant's sternum, just below the level of the nipples. The depth of compression is reduced to 1.5 inches.

103) (A) Place two fingers on the infant's sternum, just below the level of the nipples.

To perform chest compressions on infants, place two fingers on the infant's sternum, just below the level of the nipples. The depth of compression is reduced to 1.5 inches. The rate of compressions remains at a range of 100 to 120 per minute.

104) (D) Quality control.

Quality control determines that a test kit or equipment is functioning properly.

105) (C) Informing the right staff of critical values.

Only Option C is correct.

The National Patient Safety Goals of the Laboratory include:

- Two-method verification for accurately identifying the patient

- Labeling specimen containers while the patient is around
- Taking note that the patient's room number and ward do not qualify as reliable identifiers
- Efficient communication systems
- Informing the right staff of critical values
- Standard precautions to mitigate risks of infections
- Adherence to hand-hygiene protocols

106) (C) Immediately perform the test as STAT.

When a missed test has been discovered, this automatically becomes a STAT test.

107) (D) Signing your initials with the date and time of collection.

Guidelines for documenting in a patient's chart:

- Use black ink.
- Sign your initials with the date and time of collection.
- Use only standardized abbreviations (when necessary).
- Write complete documentation of your actions and patient actions.
- To correct an error on paper, draw a single line across it and sign your initials.
- To correct an error online, do not erase the previous entry; instead, enter the updated result with a comment alerting you to the new entry.

108) (A) Reduce medical errors.

In compliance with quality-management systems, laboratories are required to develop a program to manage non-conforming events. This involves identifying issues within the laboratory workflow processes and improving them to provide better patient care and ensure the safety of patients and staff. It also includes the implementation of changes to these processes and procedures. Finally, it serves to investigate and remove the causes of these nonconforming events. All these activities are aimed at reducing medical errors.

109) (A) Quality indicators.

A quality indicator is presented through graphs that measure the laboratory processes' performance.

110) (B) Six Sigma.

Six Sigma was adopted by The Joint Commission to guide laboratory facilities. Its main goal is to reduce errors to the acceptable level of 3.4 defects for every million opportunities. A laboratory that arrives at the Six Sigma level has addressed the most important variables for quality patient care.

111) (D) Failures of the process.

A root cause analysis begins with investigating and reconstructing the event's details to outline the actions that could have caused it. The analysis is meant to focus on the failures of the workflow procedures and not on the staff's mistakes

112) (D) Albumin and malnutrition.

Only Option D is correctly paired.

113) (B) Hyperparathyroidism.

Hyperparathyroidism results from the excess parathyroid hormone. This causes hypercalcemia due to excessive bone resorption. It affects the bones (pain, fractures) and causes kidney stones, lethargy, depression, and abdominal upset.

114) (D) Only A and C.

The hormone progesterone, together with human beta chorionic gonadotropin (detected in serum and urine pregnancy test kits), is increased at this time to help maintain the pregnancy.

115) (D) *Neisseria gonorrhea* (gonorrhea).

Sexually transmitted diseases cause inflammation or lesions in the genital organs. Common bacteria and their corresponding disease include:

- *Chlamydia trachomatis* (chlamydia)
- *Trichomonas vaginalis* (trichomoniasis)
- *Herpes simplex* virus (herpes genitalis)
- *Treponema pallidum* (syphilis)

- *Neisseria gonorrhea* (gonorrhea)

116) (B) Streptococcal tonsilitis.

When you have any of these, it is best to avoid contact with others until you are out of the infectious stage:

- Active hepatitis A
- Active tuberculosis
- Bacterial or viral conjunctivitis
- COVID-19 (even if asymptomatic or mild)
- Dysentery
- Flu or influenza
- Herpes zoster
- Infection with lice or scabies
- Measles
- Mumps
- Pertussis
- Streptococcal tonsilitis
- Varicella

117) (C) *Clostridium difficile.*

Of the following choices, only *Clostridium difficile* colonizes the intestines after antibiotic overuse. It is responsible for causing toxic megacolon or pseudomembranous colitis.

118) (D) Arthritis.

Arthritis involves joint pain, swelling, erythema, and warmth of the overlying skin.

119) (C) Seizure.

Seizures result from abnormal transmission of electrical impulses due to electrolyte imbalances, infections, fever (benign seizures of childhood), or traumatic injury to the brain. While it is rare, seizures may be triggered by venipuncture.

120) (A) Hepatitis B.

There are currently no effective vaccines for the following:

- Human immunodeficiency virus
- Hepatitis C
- Human T-lymphotropic virus
- West Nile virus
- *Trypanosoma cruzi*
- *Treponema pallidum*

A vaccine is available for hepatitis B. It is provided free of charge to exposed employees, as mandated by OSHA.

Made in the USA
Middletown, DE
06 June 2025